FIT – STRONG – LEAN

FIT STRONG LEAN

BUILD YOUR BEST CIRCUIT TRAINING PLAN

MIKE DIEHL

FELIX GREWE

Meyer & Meyer Sport

British Library Cataloguing in Publication Data
A catalogue record for this book is available from the British Library
Originally published as *Fitter Stärker Schlanker,* © 2018 by Meyer & Meyer Verlag

Fit. Strong. Lean.
Maidenhead: Meyer & Meyer Sport (UK) Ltd., 2019
ISBN: 978-1-78255-171-3

© 2019 by Meyer & Meyer Sport (UK) Ltd.
Aachen, Auckland, Beirut, Dubai, Hägendorf, Hong Kong, Indianapolis, Cairo,
Cape Town, Manila, Maidenhead, New Delhi, Singapore, Sydney, Teheran, Vienna
Member of the World Sport Publishers' Association (WSPA)
Printed by Print Consult, GmbH, Munich, Germany

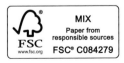

ISBN: 978-1-78255-171-3
Email: info@m-m-sports.com
www.thesportspublisher.com

CONTENTS

1 INTRODUCTION

Your body is your temple!

What is the difference between a winner and a loser? In my opinion, it is primarily one thing: self-confidence. I have been working with professional athletes, actors, and business leaders for many years. I prepare them for competitions or specific roles, helping them to create a balance in their exhausting professional lives and achieve their athletic goals. However, one thing I notice again and again is that the more successful a person is in what he does, the greater his self-confidence, self-reliance and with a few exceptions - his athletic performance capacity.

Successful people have learned to regularly overcome their inner-couch potato. They are able to do this when it comes to exercise because they have also been able to manifest this in other areas of their lives, and vice-versa. They know how to overcome mental difficulties, and their conviction that nothing and no one will stop them from achieving their goals is able to lend them the critical self-confidence required for exercise. A fit and healthy body significantly contributes to a person's ability to appear more self-confident, and therefore more successful in other areas of life than those that are overweight and experiencing health problems.

In this book, I will show you many effective and versatile exercises for your fitness training that will get your entire body into the kind of shape it may never have been in before. You will work out with your own bodyweight as well as some small aids – stability balls, resistance bands, and free weights. In addition, I will explain how you can change your attitude about exercise so radically that regular workouts will become a part of your life as much as brushing your teeth. Self-discipline is an important factor when it comes to continuously meeting new athletic challenges. In the chapter on motivation, you will learn what that means and how you can develop this ability.

Back in our first book (*Bodyweight Training mit Mike Diehl*), I compared the body to a temple. Yes, your body is your personal temple in which your soul wants to reside in good health and happiness. That also means that only you are responsible for how you take care of this temple, the home of your soul. If you allow it to decay slowly but surely, the day will come when it will no longer be inhabitable.

The following quote has shaped my life and me: *"Pain doesn't stand a chance against passion. It is about finding a goal for which you are willing to accept pain and hard work."* In my life, my athletic drive originated in my military service. As a member of the Special Forces, I had to literally train for survival and often had to fight for my life. Numerous deployments in conflict areas have changed my attitude about life and made me more aware of what is important. People living in poor countries of deployment made me realize that happiness and success are not measured by wealth, but rather satisfaction. To me there is nothing more important than self-satisfaction, and there is no doubt that the basis for this is a strong and healthy body.

When I was younger I had a major accident while parachuting and the doctors told me that I would never be able to properly exercise again. However, I was not interested in their prognosis. I was wheelchair-bound but would still find staircases in the hospital and do pull-ups on the stair-rails. My legs were incapacitated, but why shouldn't I exercise my arms and upper body? Once I was—contrary to expectations—more or less recovered, I completed my first backpack runs and returned to parachuting as quickly as possible. It was a classic case of therapeutic confrontation.

Even today I can still feel some of the pain caused by my horrific accident. However, it never stood a chance against my passion for exercise and working out. Overcoming it had nothing to do with physical abilities, but solely my attitude and love for sports.

Why am I telling you this? On the one hand, it is to illustrate the seemingly unattainable goals that people can achieve. On the other hand, it is to also make you aware that you should appreciate your body. Be happy that you have it and seize that opportunity to keep it fit and energized long-term through healthy exercise.

The workout chapter in this book is very extensive, offering many exercises with lots of variations. You will work out without apparatuses, but rather with some aids. There is, however, one thing that won't change: all of the exercises and circuits you will learn beginning on page 186 can easily be done at home. You will not need a fitness studio, and most definitely no machines. You will work out in front of the television or on the floor in your bedroom.

I am a big fan of the American KISS system – Keep it simple, stupid! In my opinion, simple workouts are the best way to success. Short and intense workouts that don't take more than 15-20 minutes per day, and without complicated exercises, are enough to bring the body up to a nice fitness level. I will therefore show you exercises that a top-athlete can use to push himself to his limit, just as much as a 40-year old homemaker or a 68-year old retiree can. Everyone works out at their own level and everyone structures his repetitions, sets, and breaks according to his own capabilities.

Only one thing is important to succeed: get the max out of every one of your workouts! How much of your potential -not just during exercise- do you think you meet on a daily basis? I'll tell you: when you think you've reached your limit, you still have a 20-30% reserve! It is often like that on the job, especially when it comes to exercise!

I hope you have lots of fun with this book and of course with your workouts. Begin by working through the individual chapters and familiarizing yourself with the exercises with the stability balls, resistance bands and free weights. At the end, you will find various circuits that are assigned a certain number of points per set. The **get fit with points system** allows you to review your performance each week or compete against your workout buddy. It is said that competition stimulates peak form.

And always remember: no one was born a pro. Anyone is able to achieve his personal goals by steadily working towards them.

Mike Diehl

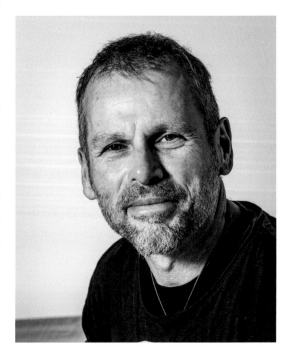

Fun is the best motivation!

I can clearly remember my first workout with Mike Diehl. I was lying on a thin towel on the dock of a Turkish beach and laboring in the hot midday sun. Bodyweight training was on the agenda. Back then, I was on an assignment as a reporter for *tennis MAGAZIN*. I submitted myself to a self-experiment with the fitness coach for the German Fed-Cup team. My incentive was to experience just how Angelique Kerber, Andrea Petkovic, Sabine Lisicki & Co. were working out.

The workout took all of 15 minutes but felt like two hours. Once it was over, I found myself lying on the floor for several minutes, almost like a boxer after a knockout punch, gasping for air and cursing my idea of training with this tough guy, who had insisted that I do pushups as a "recovery" between two exercises. Mike kept barking not to make such a fuss, making me feel like Rocky Balboa about to prepare for his final fight.

Our meeting in Turkey was the start of the ingenious idea of bringing together a workout book of Mike's exercises and philosophy. The deal was that Mike would provide the content and I would put it into the correct form, and verbalize it while also taking care of the editorial process.

Our first collaborative work appeared in March 2015. We published the book, *Bodyweight Training mit Mike Diehl*. The book was originally published in German, and it is not available in English. After this book, we published *My Fitness Journal*, a great way to record your fitness goals and training for a year. Our work fills us both with pride.

With our first book, there were unfortunately some pitfalls that occurred during the publication process. Our story can easily be applied to everyday life and athletics. All of us are familiar with setbacks. They are a part of life, so when able to understand their hidden message, they become very helpful in our personal development. As a recreational athlete, I frequently have days where it is difficult to motivate myself to work out. This is mostly when other areas of my life are particularly draining, such as when stress at work or my private life are robbing me of the necessary energy, or I am impacted by the shortness and cold of fall and winter days.

However, what I have learned in the years of working with Mike is that it is helpful to stand up against your lack of motivation, particularly during these phases. When someone doesn't perceive his regular workouts as a burden or obstacle, but rather as enrichment for one's body and an outlet for irritation and day-to-day worries, he can quickly head off motivational lows. The attitude towards exercise determines whether we fluctuate between peaks and valleys like a wave, or whether we continuously and steadily train at a high level.

For me personally, gratitude is a major motivator. For example, the fact and remembrance that I am healthy and not wheelchair-bound like many other people, the fact that I can move my arms and legs. While working together, my conversations with Mike have also shaped me in that regard. I am now more often able to think: I don't *have* to go work out. No, I am *able* to!

In the fast pace of our daily life, we often take our own health for granted. Just turning on the TV at night to watch the news is enough to become aware of the suffering and cruelty in this world. How small are our problems compared to those of people living in war-torn regions? And getting back to fitness: how grateful should we be for being able to live in an oasis like Western Europe, where at most it is laziness and the daily grind that keep us from working out?

One important lesson I have also had to learn: we can only reach our fitness goals if we integrate our fitness training into our lives so it becomes a part of us. With this book and its versatile workouts, we wish to help you do just that, and most of all, convey to you the joy of physical fitness. There is honestly no better motivation than fun and passion!

Just one last plea before you get started: we love feedback, especially on our social media platforms. Please, follow us on Facebook (/fitnesscoach.mikediehl) and Instagram (@Mike_Diehl_Training). And visit us on our website at: www.mike-diehl.de

Have lots of fun and success with your workouts!

Felix Grewe

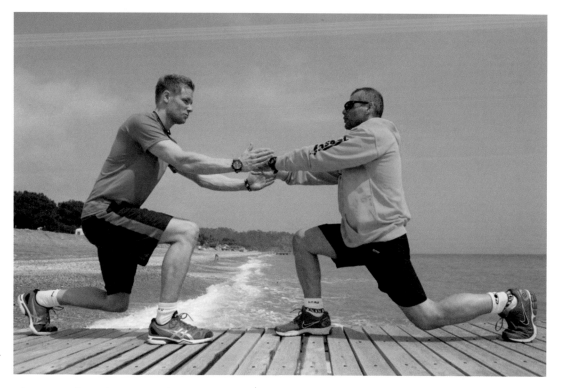

The two authors during their first joint workout in the spring of 2013, in Turkey.

Acknowledgments:

We would like to thank models, Annabell and Leslie, for their great dedication.

2 WORKING OUT WITH THE STABILITY BALL: PLAY YOURSELF FIT!

Back in our first book, I explained that working out at home using your own bodyweight is absolutely enough to reach a high fitness level and do health-oriented exercise. So why are we now using small implements like the stability ball, resistance bands, or free weights in our second book? Because they are easy to incorporate into your workouts at home. In spite of using these implements, you still do not need a fitness studio. They also add some variety. For many people, bodyweight training is an important alternative but it is not the only one. Someone who likes some variety can jazz up his workouts with small implements.

The *stability ball* was originally created as a toy in Italy in the 1960s. These balls were soon used for sports physical therapy, particularly to help treat back problems. The stability ball's unstable base forces you to use your deep muscles more to keep your balance during exercises.

The result: your core muscles get stronger, your posture more stable – the foundation for a well-supported and pain-free spine. Even seemingly easy exercises like the triceps pullover or shoulder-press with two free weights become much more difficult when you do them while lying on your back on a stability ball. You will be introduced to these exercises later.

The stability ball offers a near inexhaustible choice of exercises. It is therefore a must for versatile workouts. Many people also use it as an alternative to office chairs in order to improve their seated posture. However, studies now show that the stability ball is not better than an ergonomic desk chair. Sitting on the ball too long and without a backrest can cause an overuse of the muscles. My tip: if you don't want to give up the stability ball as an office chair, you should only use it periodically for 30-60 minutes per day.

Why work out with the stability ball?

The stability ball is well suited for athletes of all ages. There are many possible exercise variations so being able to combine them with other implements like Deuser resistance and exercise bands or free weights, can offer suitable challenges for beginners as well as pro athletes.

Another factor: working out with a stability ball doesn't just bring variety to your workout, it's also fun. Many exercises may initially seem difficult, primarily with respect to balance. But the more you integrate them into your workouts, the better you will be able to do them over time.

If you also engage in other forms of exercise that require good physical balance, you will benefit from your improved balance. However, we recommend some exercise experience and a certain fitness level as a foundation for at least the more ambitious exercises. The purchase price of a stability ball is definitely reasonable and much less than the cost of a membership at a well-equipped top-notch fitness studio.

Which ball is right for me?

Stability balls come in different sizes. Choosing the right ball therefore depends on your height.

The following guidelines apply:

< 5 feet tall = 45 cm ball

5' – 5'5" = 55 cm ball

5'6"- 6'2" = 65 cm ball

6'3" – 6'7" = 75 cm ball

6'8" and taller = 85 cm ball

Practice tips for the stability ball

1.   If you are a beginning user of the stability ball, you should first get used to the implement. Keep both feet on the floor and use a wall for stability.

2.   Advanced users should utilize the ball's possibilities and complete the exercises vigorously.

3.   Make sure your "work space," meaning your workout area, is cleared of sharp objects. Other exercise implements and furniture should be far enough away so that you won't hurt yourself if you do happen to fall off of the ball.

4.   Find out about the stability ball's maximum weight limit. Additional weights and vigorous exercises place more stress on the ball than standard exercises.

5.   Make sure your movements are always slow, clean, and controlled.

You can find stability ball exercises starting on page 65 of this book.

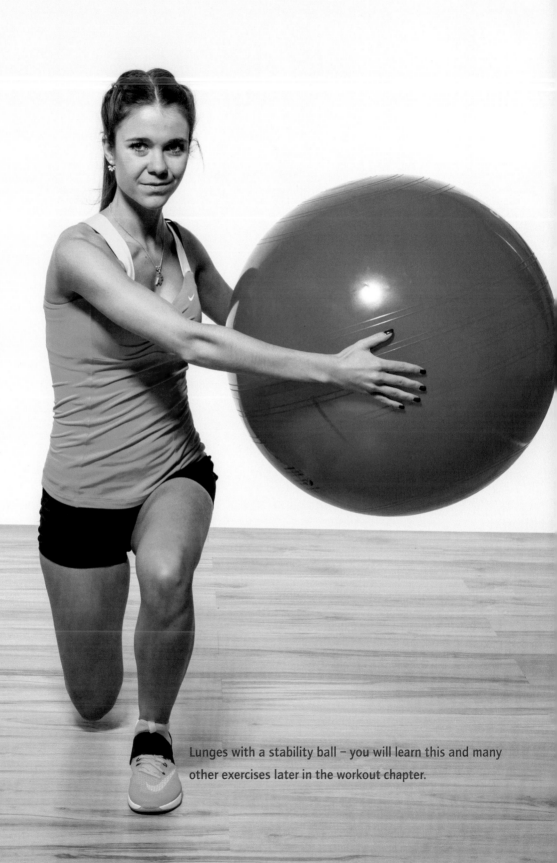

Lunges with a stability ball – you will learn this and many
other exercises later in the workout chapter.

3 RESISTANCE BANDS: THE SMALLEST PORTABLE FITNESS STUDIO

Have you ever worked out with *resistance bands*? If not, I urge you to integrate them into your workout right away, regardless of any prejudices you may have. During my time as a commander of Special Forces in the German army, I bought a Deuser band for everyone in my squad. Those tough guys were a little skeptical at first. They thought those rubber bands were only for women and targeted rehab training. Back then, I had to listen to a lot of grumbling. But I proved them wrong with the first workout unit, and no later than when the toughest guys hit their limit, did I have my men convinced. By now the bands have long found their place in the side pocket of their combat uniforms.

Exercise bands aren't just a must for soldiers. I recommend them to anyone looking for a way to work out at home, or to those wanting to complete a good workout within a short period of time. They are also great for individuals looking to stay fit during business trips or vacations, or those wanting to supplement endurance runs through the woods with outdoor strength training,

regardless of whether they are young or old, beginner or pro.

Strength training with rubber bands was developed back in the 1960s with the legendary story of when Erich Deuser trained his national soccer team with bicycle inner tubes. In 1967, he developed the circular Deuser band, which quickly became very popular and was soon used by every ambitious athlete. Today there are many types of resistance bands on the market. Different manufacturers produce them in various colors, strengths, and lengths. I personally prefer the red and blue Deuser bands because the colors signify different levels of resistance, but there are so many other resistance bands you can use.

Since I often travel around the world with my clients and athletes, resistance bands have become essential to my work. They fit into any bag, regardless of how small. They also fit beside my personal "fitness box," i.e. my own body, and provide excellent support anytime.

Why work out with resistance bands?

Of course you can accomplish a lot with just bodyweight exercises. It is common knowledge that I am a big fan of bodyweight training. But over time many athletes reach a point when effective muscle building without implements becomes increasingly difficult. Resistance bands allow you to set new, above-threshold stimuli.

Many strength-training experts consider the progressive load increase as the determining factor for muscle growth. While you can also achieve this with just bodyweight exercises, it is much more difficult than with the use of resistance bands. You can use different-strength bands and shorten your hold on the band to increase resistance, or use multiple bands at one time.

Besides, the keyword variation is an unbeatable argument. If you work out often, resistance bands are an excellent alternative, even if you regularly go to the fitness studio. No one is able to do the same exercises forever. If you complete the same program week after week, you will eventually face two significant problems: one, you will lack motivation because monotony kills pleasure. And secondly, because you will no longer notice any progress because your body has gotten used to the workout.

Optimal use of resistance bands

With a little imagination, any bodyweight exercise can be made harder with a resistance band. Even many classic exercises that are performed on machines at the fitness studio can be replicated with just one or two bands. You can find suggestions and exercises beginning on page 82 of this book.

Study results have long verified the extremely positive effects of resistance bands on health and fitness. The following effects, among others, have been verified: Increased strength

- Improved balance
- Improved posture
- Reduced pain
- Fall prevention
- Lower blood pressure
- Increased strength endurance
- Increased functionality

The steady increase of resistance during motion execution ensures that the maximum resistance occurs when the muscle is at maximum efficiency. Forgoing additional weights makes resistance-band training one of the safest types of strength training. In addition to building muscle, stimuli that improve movement coordination are also created. There are, however, critics that are skeptical about the effects or resistance bands. They believe that they don't substitute traditional weight training with heavy weights.

I suggest doing a biceps or triceps workout based on the *Tabata principle*. It is an interval method also known as HIIT training (high-intensity interval training). The ratio between athletic activity and recovery during a Tabata set is 2:1. That means you work out for 20 seconds and then rest for 10 seconds. These intervals are repeated eight times. It takes approximately four minutes to complete one Tabata set. They are, however, quite brutal.

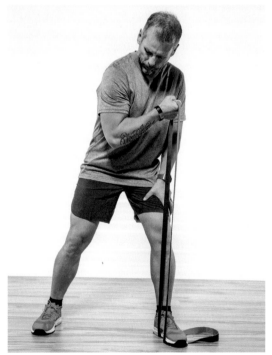

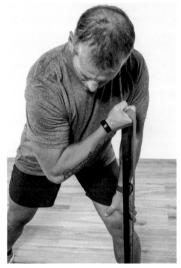

With resistance bands, you can perfectly work all muscle groups.

Practice tips for resistance bands

1.   Heavy-duty resistance bands in particular can be hard on the hands. Women are especially sensitive to this. Wear workout gloves just like many athletes do during gym workouts and free-weight training at the fitness studio.

2.   Never insert or clamp the resistance band somewhere with sharp edges or where it is able to cause damage. During most exercises, there is so much tension on the band that it can leave marks on, for instance, wooden chairs.

3.   With the right care, the band will last longer without becoming sticky. Make sure that your resistance band is always in good condition. Check it regularly and exchange as soon as you notice tears.

4.   Get over your initial skepticism and give resistance band workouts a chance. I speak from experience when I say: you will get used to it extremely fast and it won't be long before they become a regular part of your workouts. I cannot imagine my daily work with regular clients and pro athletes without the use of resistance bands.

5.   Make sure your movements are always slow, clean, and controlled.

You can find exercises with resistance bands starting on page 82 of this book.

4 DUMBBELLS: THE GATEWAY TO WEIGHT TRAINING

Free weights are generally the symbol for effective strength training and fit, hardened bodies. Everyone automatically associates them with strong muscles and sweaty workouts. I don't have to tell you that it is possible to work out just as hard and effectively without free weights. Nevertheless, free weights are considered the gateway drug to strength training, and they're not only valid but indeed also recommended implements that should occasionally be included in your workouts. Free weights in particular remind many athletes of old prison movies where inmates get pumped up with dumbbells behind bars, while decreasing their aggressions.

The image of the free weight has definitely changed since then. Even delicately built women use them regularly in their workouts.

Much like stability balls and exercise bands, free weights have three important advantages: they are inexpensive to purchase and don't take up much space, which makes them easier to use at home. They are also able to generate a considerable amount of resistance.

We differentiate between **bone dumbbells** and **barbells**. Bone dumbbells are made of one piece, and due to their construction, have the major advantage of no parts coming loose during use. By contrast, **barbells** are much more versatile. They can be loaded with more or less weight, and their use is therefore multifunctional, depending on the exercise and the athlete's fitness level. The weight can generally be varied without problem from between 3 kg and 20 kg (6.6 and 44 lbs.). Barbells are almost always available as a set with different weights.

Why work out with free weights?

Working out with free weights has many advantages. For instance, you can work individual muscles as well as different muscle groups. You can even target hard to reach deep muscles with rotational movements while also working your so-called *intermuscular coordination*, because free-weight training includes compensatory movements that combat muscular imbalances, unlike classic exercises done on many machines at the fitness studio.

On principle, I place great emphasis on functionality in my training units, particularly

when working out with free weights. Dumbbell workouts stabilize the body, predominantly the core area, the spine. This doesn't just improve overall strength, but with the correct execution of exercises, can eventually mitigate everyday conditions like back pain.

Practice tips for free-weight workouts

1. To avoid an increased risk of injury, particularly to inexperienced athletes, make sure you execute the exercises correctly.

2. Beginners should go back to basic exercises and pay attention to maintaining a stable stance, engaged abdominal muscles, and good balance.

3. Acquire either some bone dumbbells in different weights, or a set of barbells that allow you to vary the weights according to the exercise.

4. As with resistance bands, this is also true for free weights: protect your hands with workout gloves. They will prevent blisters and calluses.

5. Perform exercises that require lots of coordination in front of a mirror which will allow you to check your motion sequence and posture.

You can find free-weight exercises beginning on page 104 of this book.

5 BODYWEIGHT WORKOUTS: YOUR BODY IS YOUR FITNESS BOX

I have been working out with my own bodyweight for a large part of my life. There is a reason why we dedicated an entire book to the subject. In this book, implement-free exercises are included in many circuits. Bodyweight training covers all components of physical fitness – from strength to endurance, mobility to coordination. The combination of variety, effectiveness, and simplicity of working out without implements is unbeatable.

While it is possible to work deep muscles with the aid of exercise bands, stability balls, or free weights, the major advantage of bodyweight workouts is that you can do them anytime and anywhere. Whether you're on a business trip, on vacation, at the office, on the couch in front of the TV, or out in nature. Basic exercises like squats, pushups, crunches, lunges, dips, or jumps can be done anywhere in the world. Your personal fitness box – your body – is always with you.

On the following pages, I will provide you with detailed explanations of the most important basic exercises: **burpees**, **dips**, **mountain climbers**, **jumping jacks**, and **squats**. You will find a large selection and sensible combination of all exercises later in the workout or circuit chapter.

Why work out with your bodyweight?

Even back in my active military days, bodyweight training was the basis of physical fitness for my men and women. Whether in the field, in the barracks, or under difficult conditions during deployment abroad, I always put the boys in my squad through their paces without implements. Nowadays many competitive athletes swear by bodyweight training, and overall acceptance of workouts without implements has grown enormously in recent years. More and more people have come to realize that classic bodybuilding on machines, and with heavy iron bars in the long-term does irreversible damage to the body. It almost destroys joints and ligaments, whereas working out with one's own bodyweight is significantly healthier from a medical point of view.

Bodyweight training demands a great deal of coordination which improves *synergism*, meaning the interplay of muscles. You rarely isolate individual muscles, but instead promote so-called functional circuits, which means entire muscle groups or chains. Many exercises are so complex that they improve coordination while also working the brain.

For example, when doing pushups you immediately modify the effect by changing the position of your arm. You engage the entire core as well as arms, shoulders, and chest. You can make pushups easier by placing your hands on a step or a bench, or make them more difficult by elevating your legs, for instance on a stability ball. You will learn this ingenious and highly effective exercise later in the book.

The athlete improves his performance capacity and somatic nervous system function with multi-muscle exercises, which means optimal coordination between the brain and muscles. I call this *movement intelligence* because our reactions are increasingly intuitive and situational. At the same time, coordination is improved and the body achieves balance, thereby protecting it from injury while automatically strengthening mental abilities.

The four cornerstones of athletics

Many athletes regularly visit a fitness studio, lift heavy weight bars and move more than 100 kg (220 lbs.) on large machines. Does that make them good athletes? Definitely not! I constantly preach to my clients that they need to reconcile the different components of physical fitness with each other. These include **speed**, **mobility**, **strength**, and **endurance**.

Everyone has different strengths. Some find it easier to lift heavy free weights, while others run a half-marathon without much effort. I therefore advise you to identify your strengths and weaknesses, and then design your workouts to bring all of the cornerstones of physical fitness to a similar level. In my mind, there is no better method than bodyweight training or exercises with small implements like those you will learn later on in the book.

Running is still the most natural movement; the original movement. Regular running is –and this is scientifically proven- no longer considered the best way to stay fit or lose fat. But adding intermittent sprints (**speed**) and bodyweight exercises (**strength**) is a great way to jazz up a jog through the woods.

Balanced workouts greatly strengthen body awareness. Regular **outdoor workouts**, i.e. running combined with bodyweight exercises, aren't just fun but also promote mobility, stability, and coordination.

Burpees – the most effective whole-body exercise

Almost every athlete that works out fairly regularly is familiar with *Burpees*. Some love them; most hate them. There is no other bodyweight exercise that pushes even the toughest guys to their limit so quickly. Burpees are true all-rounders. They burn calories, improve endurance, and help to build muscle. Burpees were developed in the last century for the US Army's performance test, and today are a regular feature of all military training and physical training units that require above average physical fitness.

1

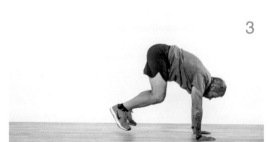

2

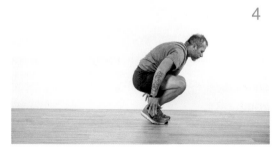

3

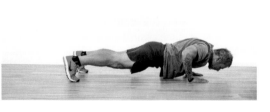

4

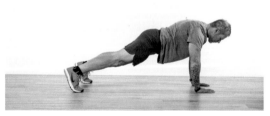

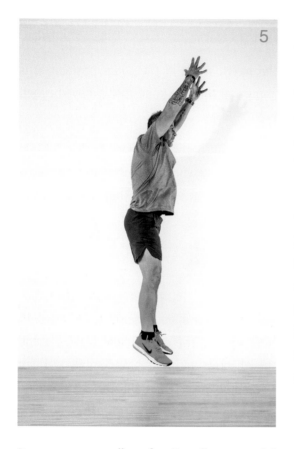

5

posture, stabilize your spine and inevitably tone the body. Burpees require lots of energy because they engage all of your muscles which means that they burn lots of calories during and even after your workout (keyword: afterburn effect), boosting fat burning long-term.

If you regularly integrate Burpees into your workout, the drudgery will definitely pay off. Hardly any other exercise is as well suited for simultaneously working on strength and endurance, improving coordination, and very quickly increasing the functional capacity of the muscles. The complex motion sequence and intense effort of major muscle groups make other exercises seem that much easier.

Burpees are excellent for Crossfit or martial arts, and are a great individual performance test for simple workouts at home or the fitness studio.

What makes those brutal Burpees so effective?

During this exercise, you use your entire body. The large muscle groups in particular, like chest, back, thighs, shoulders, and arms, are worked very intensively. Almost all areas of the body are worked simultaneously and directly. Burpees will also improve your

Squats – miracle weapon for muscle development

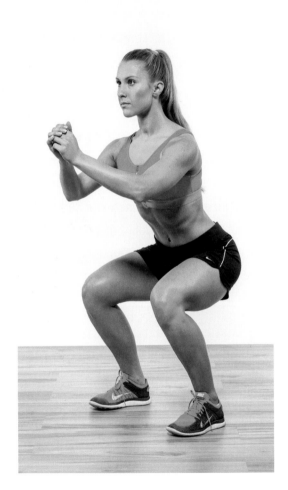

the heels. While in the squat position, it is important that the knees don't move beyond the toe line.

Women in particular tend to like squats because they work the gluteal muscles more than any other exercise. They also work the front and back of the thighs, the quadriceps and hamstring, as well as the muscles of the hips and calves.

Did you know that the muscles of the trunk, abdominals and back muscles, also benefit from squats? The erector spinae muscle and the obliques and rectus abdominis stabilize the movement and are therefore engaged during every squat. This is important, primarily because coordination and stability as well as transmission of force originate in the core, and are transferred to the entire musculature.

Many athletes underappreciate legwork – also, because the optics of muscular legs is less important to them than bulging biceps and broad shoulders. Women on the other hand, often worry that intensive training will make their legs too muscular. Nevertheless, remember that whether you want to burn fat or build muscle, leg training is indispensable! The gluteal and thigh muscles make up a large

You may remember *squats* as a warm-up exercise during PE class in school. The name squat explains the exercise during which you move into a squat from an upright standing position. The upper body is erect, eyes looking straight ahead, and the weight shifting to

portion of our overall muscle volume. Thus working these areas requires a lot of energy, and heavily stimulates fat burning. It is also similar with muscle growth. Strengthening the thighs and gluteal muscles induces an increased release of growth hormone, which promotes general muscle growth.

Are squats bad for your knees?

There are countless studies on this theory; some proving it and others disproving. Many critics also claim that the knee, due to its anatomical structure, is not well suited for the joint movement typical to squats. I, however, happen to disagree. We work our knee joints all the time, often just in our daily lives, whether this is just a suggested or lateral movement, or through bending over. The squat without weights is one of the fundamental human movements. Our joints have to be exercised, too, so that they become stronger and more resilient, allowing us to prevent injury. The more we strengthen our joints, the more synovial fluid they produce, and the better their circulation.

Let's not forget that the surrounding muscles are the most important factor in joint stability. Try to pay attention to how often you work your knees in the course of a day, for instance, having to squat to pick something up off of the floor. What matters is that you execute the movement with the correct form. Although this exercise seems simple compared to other exercises, I often see major execution errors which can certainly cause problems. You will find out how to do clean squats later on in the exercise chapter.

Climbers – mountain climbing in flat country

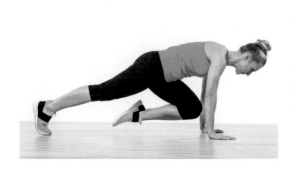

Mountain climbers are also part of the basic bodyweight-training exercises. They get their name from the movement itself, a climbing motion. You start in pushup position and alternate, moving your feet/knees towards your hands. Jumps are shallow above the floor and your bottom should not be higher than the shoulders.

This exercise may sound easy. Try it and you'll find that it can be quite brutal.

Climbers require a high level of mobility as well as explosive leg-power, while the chest and shoulder muscles have a stabilizing effect. This exercise raises the heart rate and kicks the entire metabolism to a higher level—a combination that really packs a punch.

Due to the use of different muscles and the heart rate rocketing up to a high level when the exercise is performed correctly, climbers are true fat-fighters. While the main focus is on the trunk (stomach/back) as well as legs and gluteal muscles, the muscles of the shoulders and upper arms are also enormously engaged. Climbers are considered an excellent all-around exercise and are challenging for beginners as well as pros. Push it to the limit! There is no limit to the speed and explosiveness of the leg movement.

Dips – strong shoulders, powerful arms

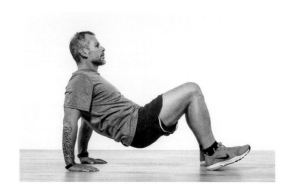

Dips are one of the fundamental bodyweight exercises that are indispensable to muscle building. They are considered one of the most effective methods for strengthening and toning the upper arms. Since the triceps on the back of the upper arm is the antagonist to the biceps, it is often difficult to work it separately in day-to-day-life. The dip motion takes place in the elbows and shoulders.

You can make the exercise more difficult by pushing off a chair, a bench, the edge of a bed or a bathtub. But dips work very well without any aids and can simply be done on the floor.

If you want to get your wish of muscular and toned upper arms, dips are without a doubt a perfect exercise you can integrate into your everyday life easily, simply, and at any time. For instance, I can recommend a *100-dips program*. It requires you to do 100 dips per day three times a week. Of course you can vary that number according to your fitness level and age. As a beginner, you should start with 30 or 50 dips. If you have already reached a high fitness level, you can even do 200 or more repetitions.

You don't need more than 30 minutes a week to strengthen your arm muscles and increase your strength. Later on in the exercise chapter, you will receive specific instructions as to which workouts will work your arms.

However, it is important to note that if you have shoulder injuries or pain, you should absolutely avoid strength exercises like dips that put a lot of strain on your shoulders.

Jacks – become a jumping jack

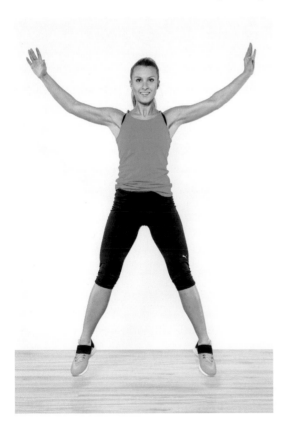

position, are extended overhead so that the hands touch. The head remains upright and the eyes should look straight ahead.

To optimally utilize jumping jacks, you need to have lots of body tension. Although nearly everyone knows of and considers this exercise to be easy, I still see execution errors all the time which can impact the effectiveness of the jacks.

Many athletes and especially trainers consider them strictly an endurance exercise, which doesn't do justice to the jumping jacks. They really work the legs, especially the calf muscles, but also the gluteus medius and minimus, as well as the inner-thigh muscles.

There are few exercises whose effects are as undervalued as jumping jacks'. You begin in a narrow upright stance and then hop into a straddle position. At the same time, the arms, which touch the side of the thighs in starting

The abdominal and trunk muscles provide the necessary stability and balance during the movement. The jumps even strengthen the muscles of the feet, which is very important for other exercises and disciplines. Even the chest, shoulder, and arm muscles are engaged. So you can truly talk about a whole-body exercise.

No doubt jumping jacks will drive up your heart rate quite a bit. Depending on the speed, jumping jacks are perfect for aerobic and anaerobic endurance training, and to increase energy consumption.

Practice tips for bodyweight training

1. Involve your environment in your workouts. When you go for a run, build in workout stations along the way where you do squats, jumping jacks, or lunges. Doing so will enhance every endurance unit and make them far more versatile.

2. Work out at the office! Yes, why not? Set aside 10 minutes out of your lunch break to complete a simple circuit. Utilize the simplicity of bodyweight workouts and the fact that you don't need any implements.

3. Alternate between strength and cardio exercises in your workout. Interval training promotes fat burning significantly more than going for a one-hour run in the woods. The Tabata principle is also a great choice.

4. Take advantage of bodyweight workouts especially at home and on the road. If you regularly go to a fitness studio, use the machines and free weights there. It will help to provide some variety.

5. To avoid incorrect movements, do the exercises slowly and with good form, rather than fast.

You can find bodyweight exercises in the various circuit workouts beginning on page 124 of this book.

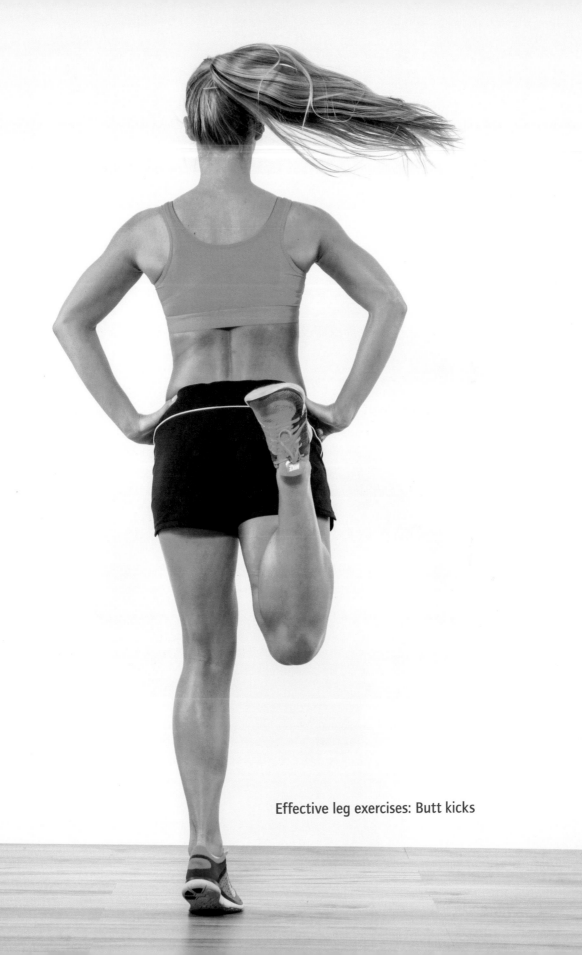

Effective leg exercises: Butt kicks

6 STRENGTH TRAINING:
CALLOMANIA VS. HEALTH

What do you associate with *strength training*? Many people think of body builders with 6-foot shoulders, pumped up iron-junkies, muscle monsters, pumpers. Most of these people do not have the experience in strength training or the valid knowledge about modern fitness training. Media reports, sometimes even in the trade press, often present a completely inaccurate picture. They show retouched dream bodies, thereby shining a spotlight on objects of comparison that will trigger feelings of inferiority in normal people and lead them to set unachievable goals. This results in quick resignation, disappointment, and frustration.

In our modern fast-paced world full of external influences, most of us struggle to escape from callomania, the obsession with beauty. Everyone pursues their personal image of attractiveness, and in doing so will often forget the uniqueness of their own body. Although we are all similar in our anatomy, our exteriors are as unique as

our thoughts and feelings about what the definition of beauty actually means.

We are constantly comparing our bodies to seemingly unachievable social ideals. Particularly as an athlete, you probably have a specific image of what the ideal upper body and legs should look like. External characteristics and our own definition of attractiveness are definitely legitimate motivators for working out. You should set well-defined and even ambitious goals for yourself. For instance, reducing fat, achieving a certain bodyweight, more toned arms, a tight butt, or building muscle mass.

But many people forget the prerequisite to achieving every goal: accepting the status quo, either of a situation or the own body. I would like to make you aware of the importance of accepting your own body, regardless of its current condition. People are rarely satisfied with what they see when they stand naked in front of the mirror after taking a shower. Few people are even halfway okay

46

with their own body, and even fewer are unconditionally happy with their looks.

Body-acceptance doesn't mean you should now be okay with a belly, flabby arms, or fat legs. No, it means that you start by acknowledging your body with its flaws and problem areas, and accept it as an important part of you. And also reconcile yourself with anatomical realities, like your height, bone structure, or hormone balance (within a healthy range!).

You should set realistic exercise goals that are in line with your physical prerequisites. No fitness training in the world will make someone who is 5'5" with a slight build look like Arnold Schwarzenegger.

Therefore, you should learn to accept your body and even love it. Set goals that can be strenuous, but are also achievable with your prerequisites. Create the best-possible version of the body that is yours today. You will be proud of yourself and suddenly view fitness training through different eyes.

Behind the glossy façade that is created by magazines, social media, and targeted marketing, you will quickly recognize the true value of strength training for a healthy body, irrespective of outer appearances and optical advantages like a six-pack or bulging biceps. Targeted fitness training primarily increases

the body's overall resilience. This means the body becomes more robust in all areas of life. I like to use the comparison of the house that rests on a more solid foundation.

Next to the muscles (active locomotor system), strength training also strengthens the passive locomotor system, the fascia, ligaments, tendons, joints, and bones. Most sports put enormous strain on the ankles, knees, and hips sometimes for several hours at a time. When the passive locomotor system has to absorb these forces alone due to a lack of stability, it increases the risk of injury.

Sprained or torn ligaments, tendonitis, or heel spurs are everyday problems shared by many recreational and performance athletes. For some athletes, a lack of core stability will also cause lots of trouble. The job of many muscles in the so-called core area is to stabilize the spine. If that is unsuccessful, the logical result often is back problems in the lumbar region.

I therefore tell everyone around me to pay particular attention to the trunk-stabilizing muscles during workouts, and not just work on strong arms and a broad back. You will learn suitable exercises in the course of this book.

Something many don't take into consideration is that contrary to the muscles that, with targeted training, often require only weeks or months for muscle growth, in other tissue types visible and perceptible changes take much longer. That means continuous training is necessary to not only bring the body in line with personal visual ideals, but most of all, to avoid injuries and long-term damages to your health.

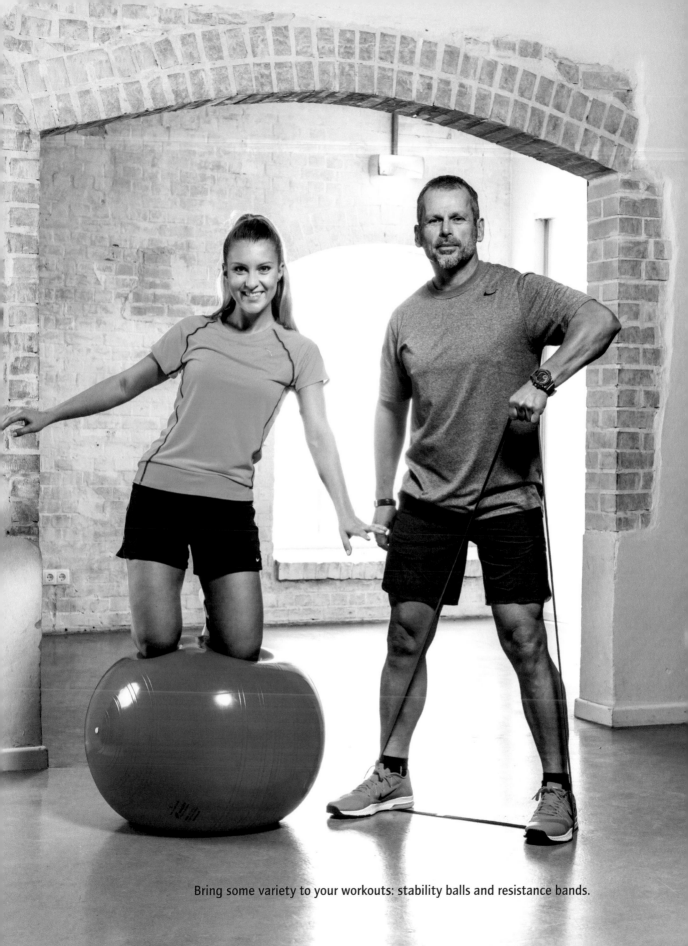

Bring some variety to your workouts: stability balls and resistance bands.

7 MOTIVATION:
PASSION WINS!

What is important to you in life? Every person defines happiness and success differently. During the years I was deployed in conflict areas with the German army's Special Forces, my priorities were limited to returning home alive and healthy. Many difficult and painful experiences have taught me to look at life as the big picture, to separate the important from the unimportant, attach less value to setbacks, and to view my existence as a precious gift. I collect brief moments of happiness every day, appreciate them, and realize time and time again that seemingly minor positive experiences in retrospect are much greater than I originally thought.

Anyone who has ever had to fear for their life or fight for survival, be it in combat or against a serious illness, ultimately tends to focus more on what's essential. We waste a lot of energy every day, getting worked up about inevitable injustices by being irritated with other people, brooding about the past, and worrying about the future. Rarely do we live in the here and now.

The fact is that thoughts are the biggest energy robbers. They deplete us like vampires; they destroy our stream of life. And yes, they keep us from achieving top performances, even in athletics. You should know that you are only able to access a fraction of your performance capacity when you are angry or stressed and worrying about problems during a workout. At the same time, the person that focuses strictly on his workout is more resilient and far more persevering.

Exercise has influenced me and my life and for many years. It has shaped my personality and character and has made me what I am today. I learned early on to view my daily workout as an opportunity for wellbeing and not an insurmountable obstacle. This has made exercise my greatest passion. I love to start the day with a good workout. Only very rarely do I see it as a burden, and

I usually feel deep gratitude for being able to wear myself out and test the limits of my physical abilities. Fortunately, I learned a long time ago to edit out any disruptive thoughts.

Unlike me, you won't have to make life-and-death decisions on a daily basis. And my attitude about exercise may seem much too extreme for your taste. Nevertheless, going forward you should try to view exercise as a helpful tool to improve your sense of wellbeing and create a foundation for a long and healthy life.

And I would ask you to internalize the following rule: whatever you do, do it with maximum love and passion! Exercise is no different than your job or your private life. An activity will only be successful if you engage in it with absolute commitment. For your daily workout this means if you learn today to feel gratitude and joy in exercise, you will be able to achieve all of your realistic goals.

Get out of your comfort zone

I have often experienced the difficulty of approaching goals, sticking with a long and arduous training program, and finishing it. Laziness and complacency always try to slow us down. And all of us ultimately have a vast repertoire of excuses to draw on. We find excellent reasons why we can't work out today—it's too hot, too late, the stomach is too empty, we have an important appointment, there's a suspenseful thriller on television, or our favorite sports team is playing—and that we'll definitely shift it into high gear tomorrow.

No matter how many motivational books and magazines you have read, or how many motivational coaches you have listened to, you are probably like the 90% of people who,

after initial enthusiasm, land back in their comfort zone. The critical quality to avoid these rollercoaster rides long-term is called *self-discipline*. If you acquire and preserve this, it will be the key to lasting success. One of my most important guidelines as a coach is that self-discipline is one of the most important qualities in people and should never be lost! Not after one week of training, not after a month, or a year.

I consider self-discipline to be one of my major strengths, and yet I am not permanently immune to setbacks. That is why ages ago, I developed four guidelines that have become imprinted on my brain like a tattoo and that you, too, should permanently internalize:

1. No one was born a professional!
2. Leave your comfort zone every day!
3. Train hard and always push your personal limits!
4. Training never ends!

The importance of self-discipline

I have been focused on the subject of *self-discipline* for decades, and it has cost me clients, lots of sweat, tears, and pain, but also joy and satisfaction in learning what self-discipline really means.

There are countless definitions and I stopped trying to count them, much less read them, long ago. Ultimately it is up to every person to find his or her own individual definition of the term self-discipline. To some, it means getting up in the morning for an early workout, walking the dog while it rains or storms, or going to a job they dislike. Others expect themselves to jog everyday, complete annual marathons, forgo certain foods, or resist a long-time addiction. Others again find strength in meditation, but in their daily lives rarely find the time to truly rest.

Our own discipline determines whether we set firm goals that involve activities or tasks that either cannot be avoided or require us to overcome obstacles, and are sometimes arduous, but ultimately good for our bodies.

I define self-discipline as the ability to always be aware of one's own strength in spite of bitter setbacks in life, in spite of social crises, blows of fate, lack of motivation, the daily grind, and feeling powerless. Never stop believing in yourself. My daily dose of exercise, usually a lengthy Krav Maga workout, helps me to remember this definition and to hold my ground every day.

If you have faith in yourself, in your abilities and your self-discipline, you will over

time be filled with a sense of invincibility, in your private life as well as your job or your sport. Achieving your goals and overcoming obstacles along the way fills you with such pride and such inner strength that going forward, you will always feel the urge to meet new and bigger challenges.

Angelique Kerber is a great example for the link between self-discipline and self-confidence. For years, "Angie" was ranked in the low mid-range among the 100 best female tennis players in the world. Anyone interested in tennis has heard all of the stories in the press about how she nearly ended her career in 2011. Angie scored one first-round defeat after another. However, she began to doubt her talent and more particularly, her mental abilities.

With a fighting spirit and especially brutal fitness training, she managed to get on the winning track. And although she was almost continuously ranked in the top 10 of the world rankings, during the years after her breakthrough, she was still plagued by self-doubt. For a long time, she stood in her own path to the big win. That is until 2016. Her triumph at the Australian Open when she beat Victoria Azarenka, whom she had not been able to beat before, and then played the match of her life against Serena Williams in the final, changed her as an athlete. Her success in Melbourne virtually pumped her up with self-confidence and was to lay the foundation for all subsequent wins alongside her jump to first place in the world rankings in the fall of 2016.

I worked with Angie for a long time, occasionally prepared her for important tournaments, or over the winter for the upcoming season. Now, when we are on the road during the Fed-Cup, I see a completely changed athlete who trusts in her own strength and draws much of her self-confidence from her superior fitness level. Angie may well be the fittest tennis player in the world, but hardly anyone possesses as much self-discipline as she does.

The four cornerstones of self-discipline

I divide self-discipline into four cornerstones. They help to make us aware of its relevance, and to integrate it into our own life instead of perceiving it as something purely abstract.

Cornerstone 1 - Acceptance

I already touched on the importance of acceptance in chapter 6, *Strength training: callomania vs. health*. Being aware of reality, acknowledging our problem areas and analyzing which mistakes led to which circumstances, is referred to as body inventory.

The amount of discipline we can muster in different areas of life varies. I know successful business people, some even upper-level managers, who pursue their professional goals systematically and with enviable focus. But they fail to optimize their lifestyle, to have a healthier diet, and to build even a minimum of exercise into their synchronized weekly schedule. On the other hand, there are plenty of examples of people that torture themselves every day in their workouts like pro athletes, but are unable to gain any footing in their job.

Accepting a condition is one of the critical steps to building self-confidence long-term. Because one thing is for sure, people who lack inner acceptance hide in either ignorance or denial. Many extremely obese people that may be dragging themselves through life can also find it easy to ignore and deny their condition.

Even in harmless everyday situations, their bodies may send signals of being overloaded such as their knees hurting while climbing stairs or their heart working too hard after a short walk. Instead of facing the critical situation and working on health-focused goals with professional help, they may resort to taking the elevator or the car. For some, they don't want to acknowledge their obesity and the likely long-term effects.

You should be aware of one thing, even if accepting truth makes you feel bad, it is your first step towards building long-term self-discipline. Regardless of what your current problem areas may be, when you learn to accept your status quo, you will incrementally gain strength and pride. In the army, we lived by these words of wisdom which I often pass on to my clients even today: To become strong you must know your weaknesses!

It doesn't matter if you already exercise regularly, have an attractive body or struggle with major weight problems. It also doesn't matter if you are in your early 20s or late 50s. My advice to you, and to every athlete I work with is that before you start a new workout phase, check your status-quo state! Only then should you set specific goals and make a plan for how you want to achieve them.

To practice acceptance of your body, I suggest you regularly ask yourself the following questions. Preferably write down the answers so you can occasionally compare them. This will help you monitor your progress.

- How do you feel at this moment physically and mentally?
- When you stand naked in front of a mirror, how do you rate your body on a scale from 1 (Pillsbury Doughboy) to 10 (Mr./Ms. Universe)?

- How often do you exercise?
- How intense are your workouts?
- Do you work out until you reach your limit? Or do you often give up when it gets uncomfortable?
- How much do you focus on your diet? How consciously do you choose what you consume each day?
- What exercise and physical goals do you pursue?
- How far away are you from achieving your goals (ideal weight, muscle mass, percentage of body fat, your times when you run, etc.)?
- How long do you think it will take you to reach your goals? And how often do you have to work out to do so?
- What is your definition of self-discipline?
- Do you consider yourself self-disciplined?
- Did you answer these questions honestly?

Cornerstone 2 - Willpower

Mahatma Gandhi once said: "Strength does not come from physical power, but from indomitable will." And the former US football coach Vince Lombardi is credited with this quote: "The difference between successful people and others isn't a lack of strength or a lack of knowledge, but a lack of will."

Both sayings have shaped and accompanied me for a long time. What is *willpower*? It is similar to defining self-discipline or acceptance; each person must find his own definition. To me willpower is the ability to focus on a goal or an activity. It is the essence of self-discipline.

Of course no one is able to muster 100% willpower for something every day and constantly, especially not exercise because the body gets tired. Fluctuating motivation is normal even after you have integrated workouts into your daily schedule for a long time, and even if you are one of those fitness junkies that are actually addicted to hard workouts.

There are always phases –sometimes hours, sometimes days, or even weeks or months- when we struggle to pursue our goals. But the more intensively you deal with the subject and realize the importance of willpower, the more you will feel the motivation it will doubtlessly give you. You will recognize your willpower when your mind calls out these beautiful words to you: "Come on, let's go!" and you feel that it is time to complete your daily workout.

In moments like these, we often put the brakes on ourselves because we don't seize the moment and instead laze around on the couch. Always remember that willpower is a resource that is often only available to us for a short time before it wanes again like the ocean during low tide.

In the military, we refer to three phases that can easily be applied to exercise:

1. Choosing and specifying a goal.
2. Making a plan of attack.
3. Executing the plan.

You summon all of your energy and position yourself for a targeted jump ahead, be it for a short 15-minute training unit that will help you feel better than you did before, or a thorough workout that will take a little longer. Always activate your willpower before your workout. To do so, be aware of your specific goals and the plan you made to achieve them. And then you execute it and apply the energy you have. You will feel your body thanking you as you work out.

Cornerstone 3 – Hard work

Many people tend to take care of seemingly easy things and problems in their lives first, putting off the more difficult work. Each of us knows how *tough* it is to tackle unpleasant tasks. We all live in our comfort zones, with some of us being able to step outside of it more easily and quickly than others.

I have a policy to help me with that, which I have committed to my brain again and again for decades: hard work is the path to success! Going on a more or less strict diet for a few weeks is relatively easy. You realized that you are putting on more fat on your hips and legs, so you pull the ripcord and eat more raw food and less sugar. Definitely, without a doubt, a good approach. But it is rarely successful in the long-term. Millions of people rely on brief diets but do so without making long-term changes to their lifestyle and changing certain habits.

This requires a certain toughness, and strong willpower. This policy applies to exercise too. At the beginning of the year, people stream en masse to the fitness studios and buy memberships to finally adhere to those good intentions of getting more exercise. They are usually the ones that stick it out for a couple weeks, generally just completing alibi workouts that are rarely challenging and don't push them to their limits.

I already mentioned in my first book that I absolutely can't stand half-hearted workouts. Keep reminding yourself that only hard work, arduous training units, and at the same time abstaining from disease-causing stimulants –this also includes excessive consumption of sugary foods- will allow you to reach your goals long-term. Make hard work your ally, not your enemy. It is not an annoying constraint, but will increasingly inspire you and make you proud as you begin to notice the results.

Passion makes hard work seem much easier. Look forward to your workout units, to afterwards getting in the shower completely drenched with sweat, to feeling all of your muscles. What is better than relaxing on the couch or the bed in the evening after a tough workout, feeling incredibly proud of your performance? Your attitude will determine whether you choose a path that is really tough and also feels that way, or choose the same path which suddenly seems much less intimidating.

Cornerstone 4 – Perseverance

There is a simple formula that can be applied to life both in general and in exercise in particular. The more *perseverance* you have, the more successful you will be! And the more successful you are, the more motivation you will have. A beautiful circle!

If you struggle with being overweight and are now starting to exercise regularly and simultaneously optimize your eating habits, you will experience this effect firsthand. In the beginning, you will struggle to stay motivated after those first training units because you won't see those pounds immediately melt away after a strenuous workout. During this phase, your perseverance will determine whether you will continue to pursue your goals or give up and indulge in your bad but familiar habits.

If you stick with it, you will soon not only feel the results, but also be able to see them. That's the moment when your motivation will automatically continue to increase.

Perseverance means diligence and endurance – no matter which area of life it pertains to. I define it as the ability to pursue a goal, to do whatever I can to achieve it, to absolutely not get emotionally distracted, and to never allow myself to be defeated by my inner couch potato.

But to me perseverance also means keeping an eye on my entire sphere, taking care even of seemingly small and unimportant tasks on my to-do list like cleaning, picking up, answering email. To me self-discipline and perseverance are part of my "way of life."

But I also want you to be able to separate stubbornness from perseverance. Because the latter doesn't mean that you can never give up. Sometimes it makes sense to change paths and adjust plans so as not to chase after an unachievable goal. Young athletes often pursue their dream of a professional career. They sacrifice their youth, train hard every day, and often realize themselves that they are not cut out for a life as a high-performance athlete. Self-discipline also means to always question whether the path you are on is the right one for you. Or whether you are pursuing a goal you are not willing to let go off solely to make your parents or friends proud.

Practice tip for self-discipline

Set specific times for important tasks. While you should keep some flexibility in your life, it is best to have some regularity, particularly with respect to exercise or small, unpleasant obligations. That means setting specific workout days and plans for when you will do which workouts—for instance circuits from this book—and how often you want to repeat them. Planning for some electronics-free time and turning off the computer and television can also be helpful. You will be in the here and now, and learn to appreciate these quiet moments and gather energy for that next workout.

8 THE EXERCISES

Enough preparation! It's time to get started. We'll begin the workouts together. First, you will learn the most important stability ball exercises. They are marked with one (easy), two (medium difficulty), or three (difficult) stars depending on the degree of difficulty. Next comes exercise, or resistance-band training, followed by free-weight training, and finally bodyweight training.

You will learn different programs that can be completed anytime, anywhere in a minimal amount of time. You will work every muscle group in your body and improve your strength while simultaneously working on your endurance, flexibility and mobility.

And finally, we will show you various circuits consisting of previously presented exercises. These have been assigned various point values according to their degree of difficulty. Your goal should be to collect as many points each week as possible. By doing so, we give you absolute control of your training. To find out how the Point-yourself-fit system works, you can turn to pages 186-187 of this book.

You can also put together your own training program with these exercises. There is no limit to the possibilities. You decide how hard you want to work out, for instance with shorter or longer breaks. To people who already possess a good basic fitness level, I recommend forgoing any breaks between exercises since you alternate muscles.

A circuit rarely takes longer than 15 minutes to complete but is a highly intense quarter of an hour during which you will physically exhaust yourself. Beginners can take occasional short breaks according to their fitness level. You can also vary the number of repetitions or the duration of an exercise according to your performance level. I generally suggest 30 seconds per exercise; however, you can start with 10 seconds, 15 seconds, or 25 seconds, and even go 40 seconds or longer. Specific suggestions will follow later on when circuits are explained.

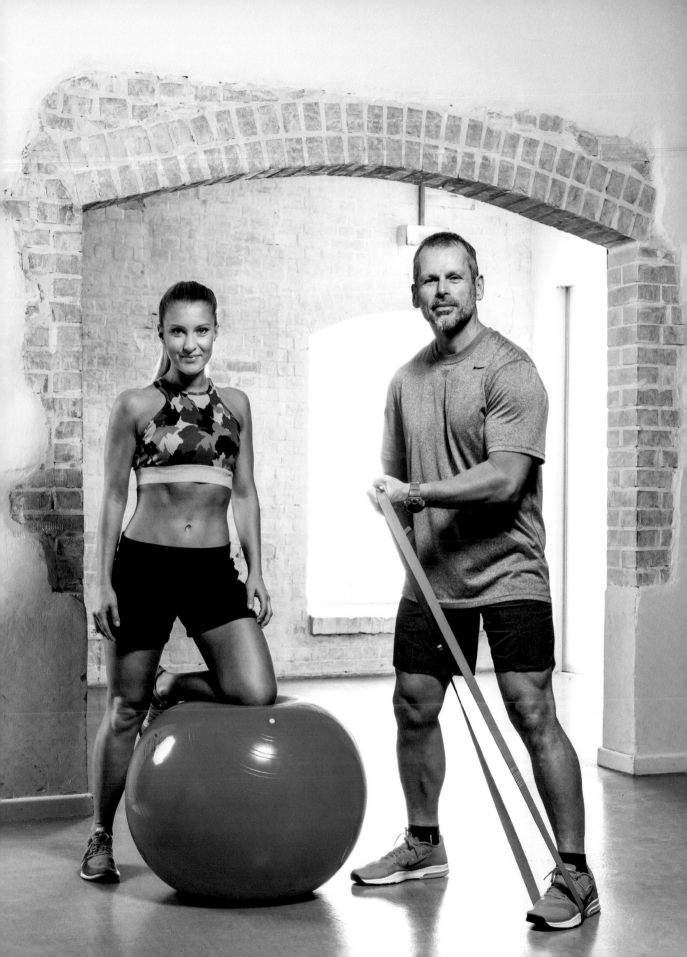

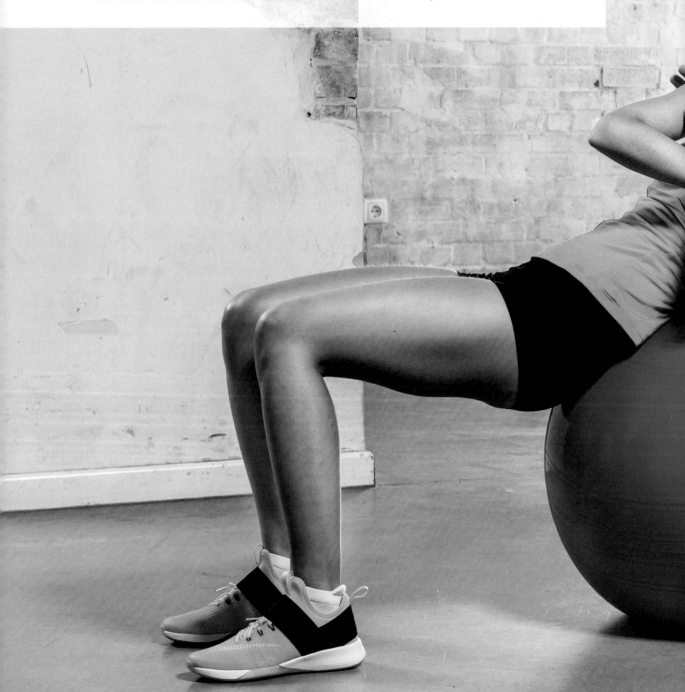

Stability ball workouts

A *stability ball* will bring some variety to your workout. You work the entire body and engage various muscles simultaneously. On the following pages you will learn the best exercises.

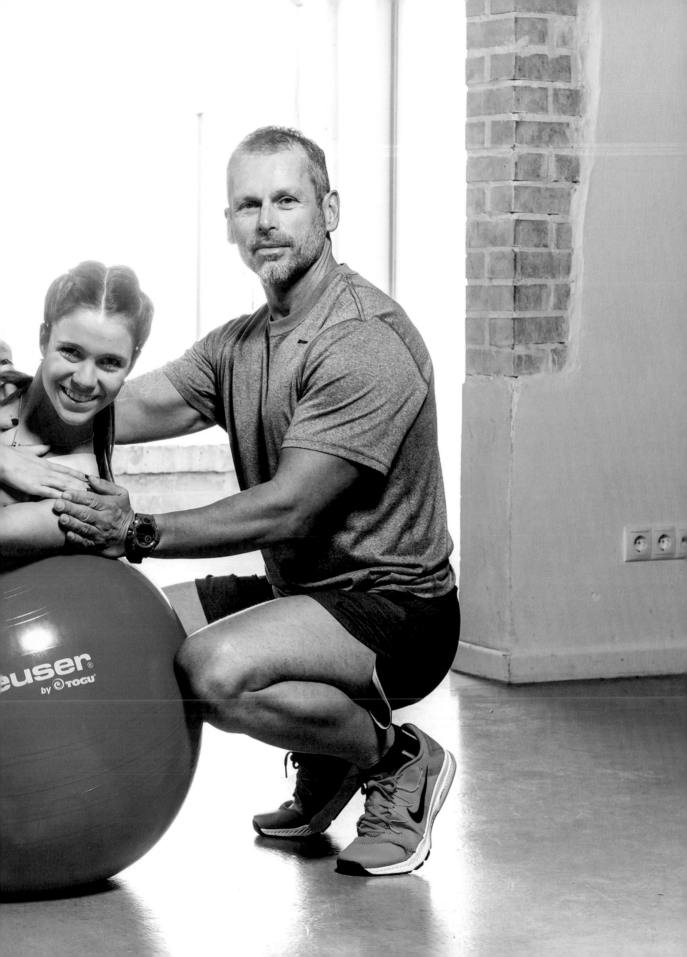

Lateral ball raise ✱✱

Gluteal muscles, obliques

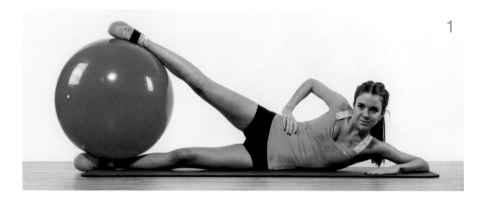

Photo 1: To start, lie on your side resting on your forearm. Hold the ball between your feet.

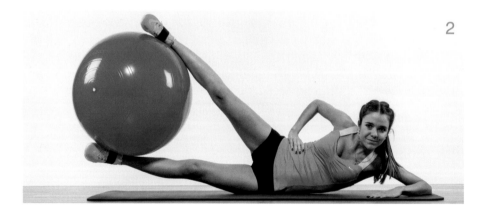

Photo 2: Now slightly raise your legs and hip, maintaining body tension. Make sure your hip stays forward. Hold this position for a few seconds and then slowly lower legs and hip.

Pro version:

Don't rest your legs on the floor. After completing one set with the appropriate number of repetitions, switch sides.

*(Asterisks indicate degree of difficulty * = easy, ** = medium difficulty, *** = difficult)*

Ball-roller ✳✳

Rectus abdominis, hip flexors

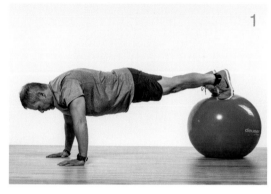

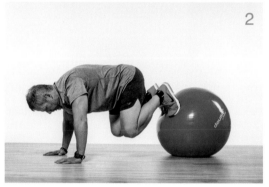

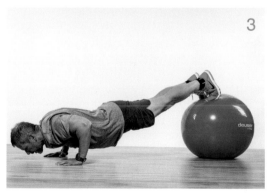

Photo 1: Begin by lying on your stomach on the ball and then roll yourself forward until only your feet have contact with the ball. Walk the arms forward and remain fully extended. Brace yourself with your hands against the floor with your shoulders vertically stacked over your arms. Pay attention to your body tension, especially in the abdominal and gluteal areas. The upper body should form a straight line and never sag.

Photo 2: Now pull the ball toward you with your feet by bending at the knees and hip joint. Hold this position for a moment, and then return to the starting position by extending your legs and rolling the ball backwards.

Photo 3: **Pro version:**

Add one or more pushups between repetitions—brutal!

Pushups on the stability ball ✳✳✳

Chest, shoulders, arms, abdominals

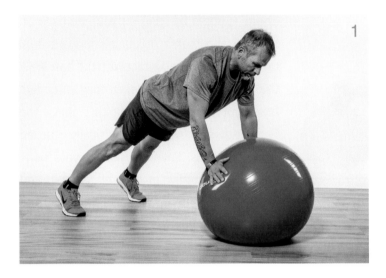

Photo 1: Get in a classic pushup position. Brace your hands against the ball with your fingers pointing to the outside. Keep your core and leg muscles engaged and your body in a straight line.

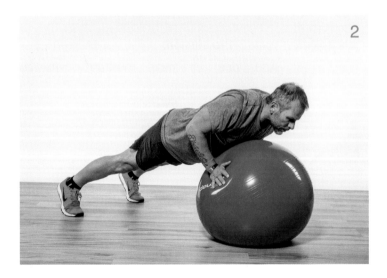

Photo 2: Now execute the pushups. Bend the elbows, lowering your sternum towards the ball. Then push back up into starting position.

Russian Twist on the ball ✳✳

Core muscles, body stability, coordination

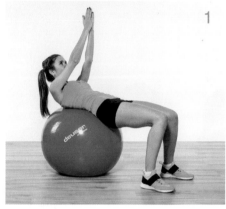

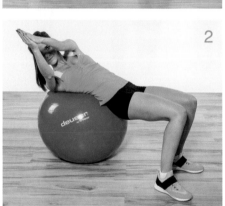

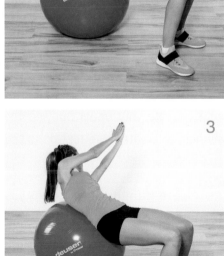

Photo 1: Lie on your back on the ball, plant your feet slightly more than shoulder-width apart, and bend the knees 90 degrees so your upper body forms a bridge with the ball. Maintain tension in your hips and bring your arms together over your head.

Photo 2: Now twist your upper body to one side with your arms extended over the shoulder. As you do so, keep your legs and pelvis steady.

Photo 3: Next, return to the starting position and then twist to the other side. You should do this exercise continuously, alternating sides.

Rotational lunge with the ball ✳✳

Thigh muscles, core

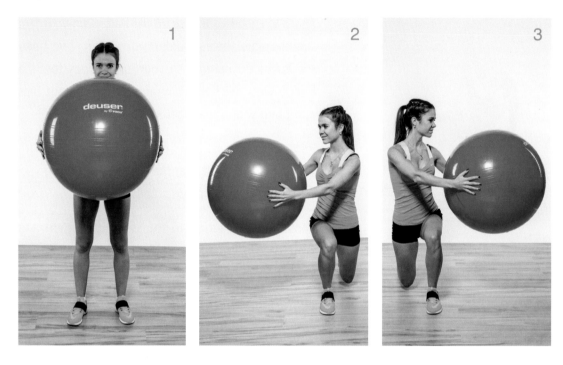

Photo 1: Stand with your feet shoulder-width apart and hold the stability ball with your arms extended forward.

Photo 2: Now execute a classic lunge: your left knee almost touching the floor and your right thigh at a 90° angle to the lower leg. Simultaneously rotate your upper body to the right. Holding the ball with your arms fully extended will help to create more tension in the shoulders.

Photo 3: Return to the starting position and now execute a lunge with the other leg. As you do so, rotate your upper body to the left.

Jackknife with the ball ✳✳✳

All of the trunk muscles, adductors, abductors, shoulders

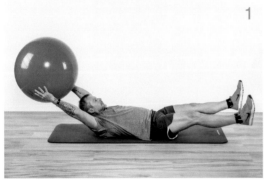

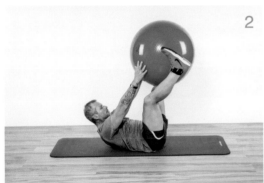

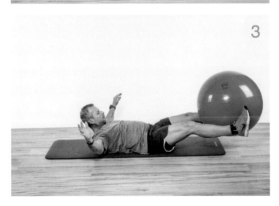

Photo 1: A brutal exercise, especially for the abs. Begin by lying on your back. Hold the stability ball above your head with your arms fully extended, and slightly raise your shoulders off the floor. Raise your feet a couple of inches as well. Please note that you should maintain high body tension!

Photo 2: Now simultaneously raise your arms and legs – the motion is reminiscent of a jackknife. Hold the ball between your calves.

Photo 3: Now slowly return to the starting position.

Double leg raises *

Lower back

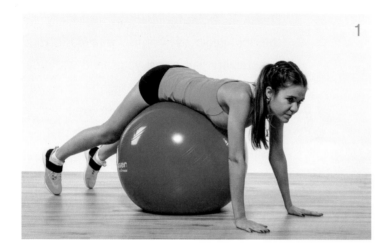

Photo 1: Lie on your stomach on the ball. Initially stabilize your body with your arms and feet on the floor, as demonstrated in the photo.

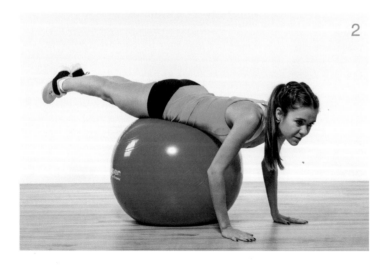

Photo 2: Now raise both legs until they are parallel to the floor while keeping the muscles in your lower back and buttocks engaged. The legs and upper body should form a straight line. Then lower your legs back to starting position. Make sure the movement is controlled.

Single leg raises ✳✳✳

Core muscles, iliopsoas muscles, shoulders

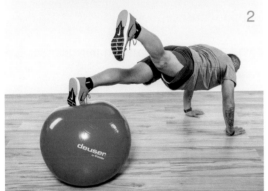

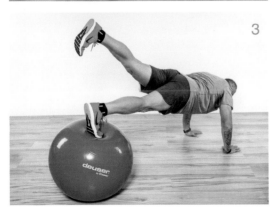

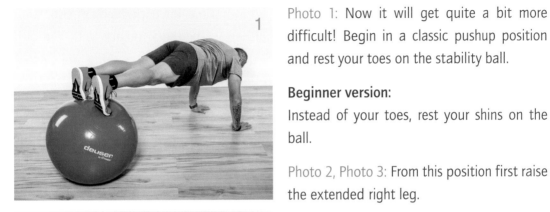

Photo 1: Now it will get quite a bit more difficult! Begin in a classic pushup position and rest your toes on the stability ball.

Beginner version:
Instead of your toes, rest your shins on the ball.

Photo 2, Photo 3: From this position first raise the extended right leg.

Please note: hold steady and maintain body tension. The ball can easily roll away. Then return to the starting position and perform the same motion with the left leg.

Partner squat ✳✳

All upper-thigh muscles

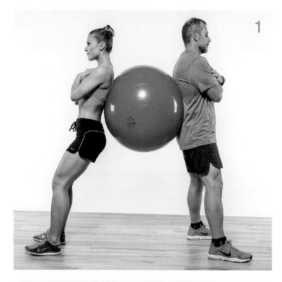

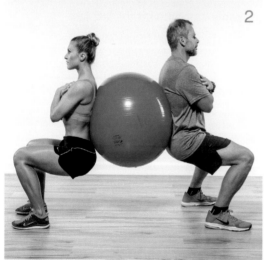

Photo 1: Time for a partner exercise. Both partners stand back-to-back with the ball held between their backs. Arms are crossed in front of the chest.

Photo 2: Now both partners do a classic squat until the upper legs are at a nearly 90-degree angle to the lower legs. Briefly hold this position and then return to the starting position. Continue by repeating this motion sequence.

If you don't have a training partner, you can use a wall instead.

Ball plank **

Abdominals, lower back, shoulders

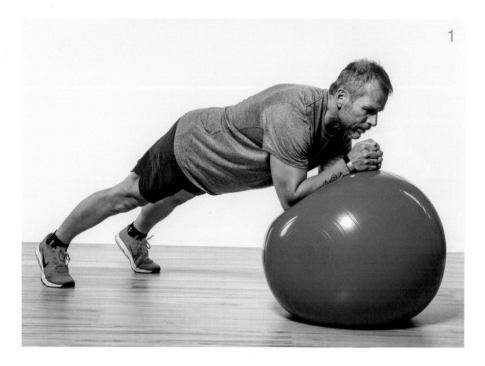

Photo 1: Brace yourself with your forearms against the ball and maintain whole-body tension with your legs fully extended. Hold this position for 20-60 seconds.

Forward ball-roller ✳✳

Abdominals, lower back, iliopsoas muscles

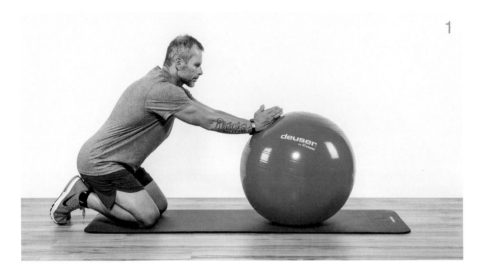

Photo 1: Kneel on the floor and sit back on your heels. Bring your palms together and place the edges of the hands on the ball with the arms fully extended, as shown in the photo. Keep your back straight.

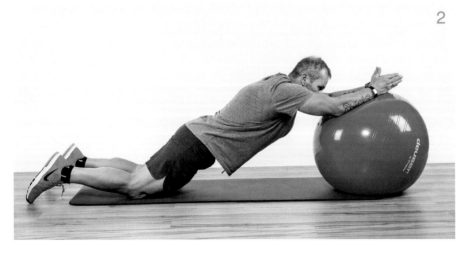

Photo 2: Now roll the ball forward until you feel lots of tension in your abs. Briefly hold this position and then return to the starting position while maintaining body tension.

Side knee-raise with pushup ✳✳✳

Whole-body exercise

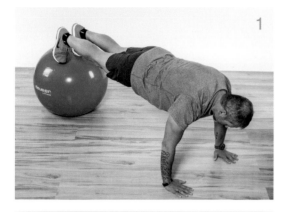

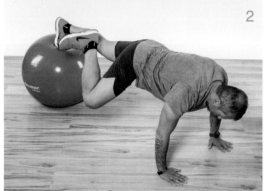

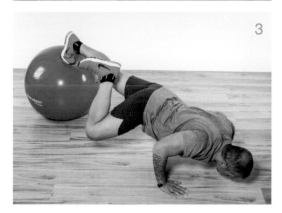

Photo 1: A brutally difficult exercise! Begin in a classic pushup position and rest your feet on the ball.

Photo 2: Now take the right foot off the ball and move your knee as close as possible to the right elbow.

Photo 3: Hold this position as you do one pushup. After you push up, straighten the right leg and place that foot back onto the ball. Next perform the same movement with your left leg.

Ball crunches ✳

Abdominals

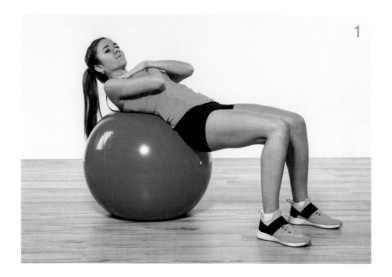

Photo 1: This is a pretty easy but effective exercise. Lie on your back on the ball with your feet planted on the floor. Cross your arms in front of your chest.

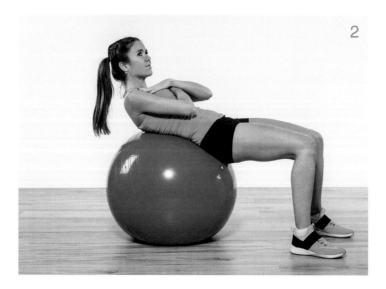

Photo 2: Now raise your upper body a couple inches while engaging your abdominal muscles, and then lower it back down. Continue this motion sequence.

Ball squat ✳✳

All thigh muscles, shoulders

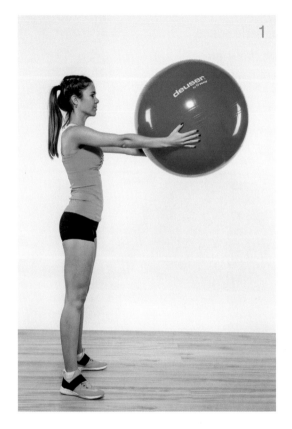 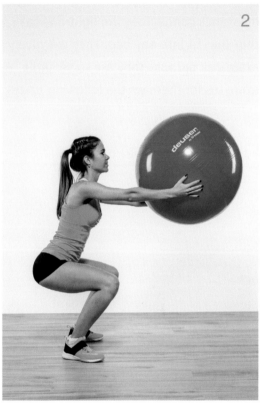

Photo 1: Stand with your feet shoulder-width apart and hold the ball with your arms extended in front of the body.

Photo 2: Now do a classic squat until your upper legs are at a 90-degree degree angle to your lower legs. The position of your arms and the ball should not change.

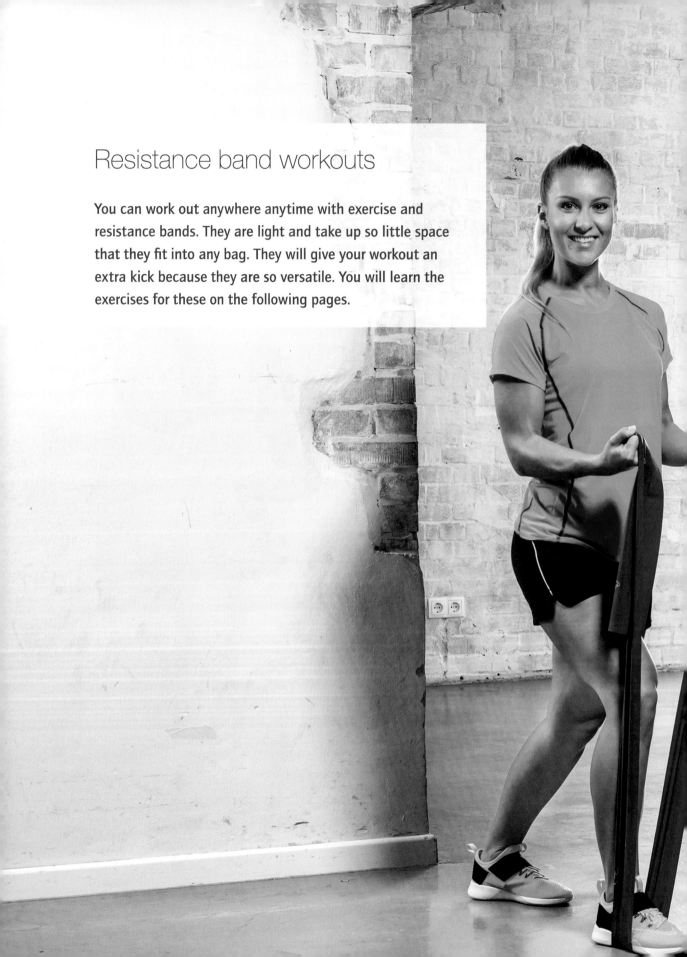

Resistance band workouts

You can work out anywhere anytime with exercise and resistance bands. They are light and take up so little space that they fit into any bag. They will give your workout an extra kick because they are so versatile. You will learn the exercises for these on the following pages.

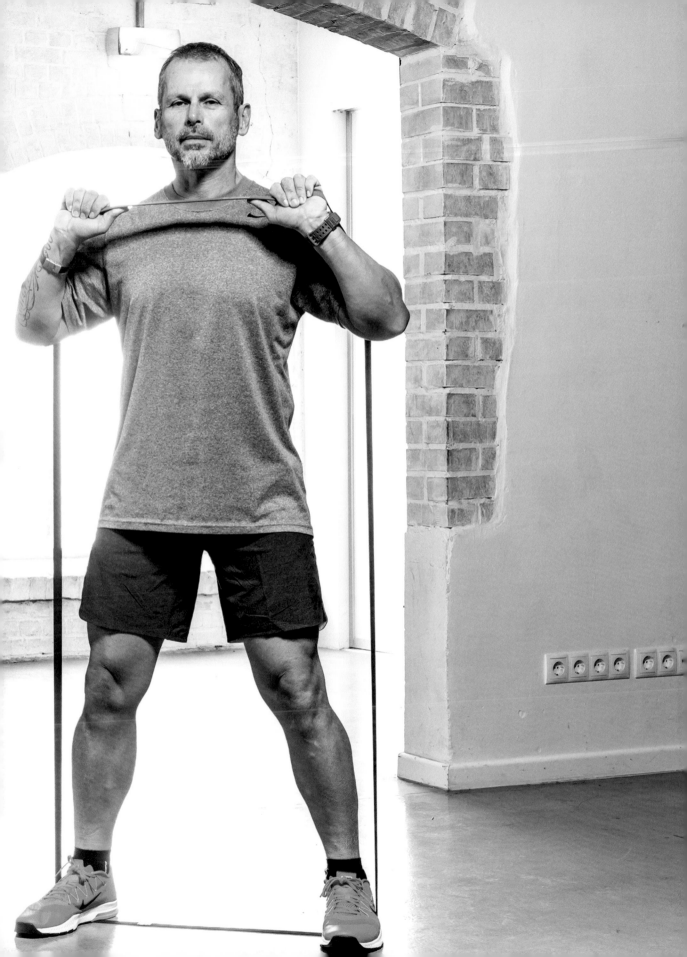

Single arm shoulder-press ✳✳

Shoulders, chest, triceps

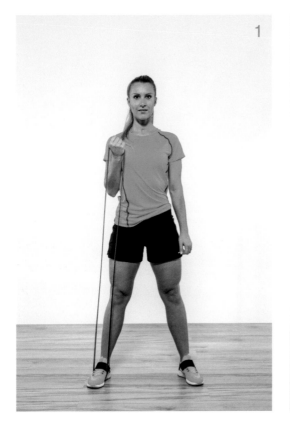
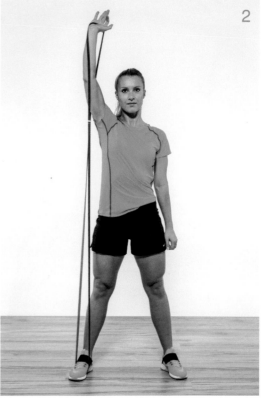

Photo 1: Stand with your feet slightly wider than shoulder-width apart. Hold the band down with one foot, grip the other end in your hand as shown in the photo and hold that hand at shoulder level.

Photo 2: Now press the band up over your head until your arm is almost fully extended. Make sure your movement is slow and controlled. Then return the arm to the starting position. Keep repeating this motion sequence.

Overhead press **

Shoulders, triceps

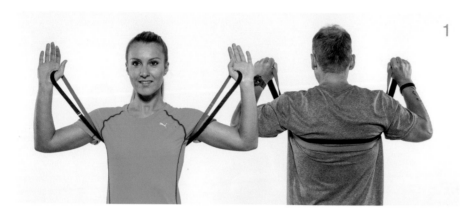

Photo 1: Place the band across your back just below your shoulder blades, and under your arms to the front of the body. Hold your upper arms in a horizontal position and bend your elbows so your forearms are at a right angle to the upper arms, as shown in the photo. Place the loops between the thumb and forefinger, making sure you have a stable, shoulder-width stance.

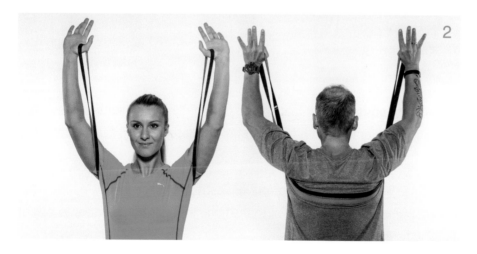

Photo 2: Now move your arms up so that your hands in their final position are above and to the side of the head. Next return the arms to the starting position. Keep repeating this motion sequence.

Squat with shoulder press ✳✳✳

Shoulders, legs, triceps

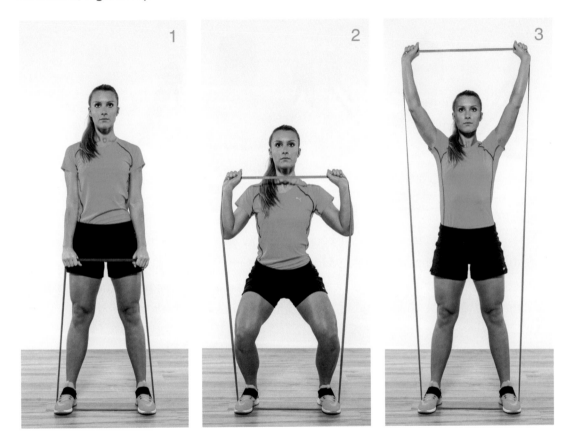

Photo 1: Start in an upright position. Your feet should be slightly more than shoulder-width apart. Hold the band on the floor with both feet, and hold the other end in front of the body with both hands.

Photo 2: Now move into a slight squat and keep your back straight. Place tension on the band by holding it at chin level. The elbows should point to the floor. Your position is similar to that of a weightlifter just before he does a barbell press.

Photo 3: Now straighten up and completely extend your arms and legs. The band now forms a rectangle and has lots of tension on it. Hold this position for two seconds and then return to the starting position.

Upright row ✳✳

Shoulders, trapezius, arms

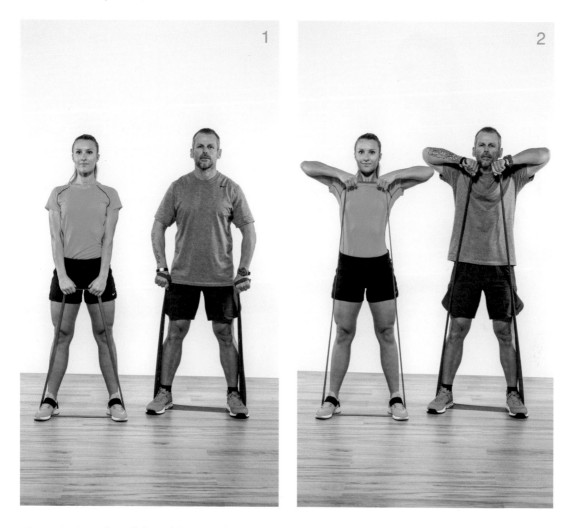

Photo 1: Stand upright with your feet shoulder-width apart and both feet on the exercise band. Hold the band with both hands, with your arms hanging loosely at the front of the body (see photo).

Photo 2: Now slowly and steadily pull your arms towards your chin. In the final position, the elbows are at shoulder-level, pointing to the outside. Return your arms to the starting position. Keep repeating this motion sequence.

Standing chest press ✳✳

Shoulders, chest, triceps

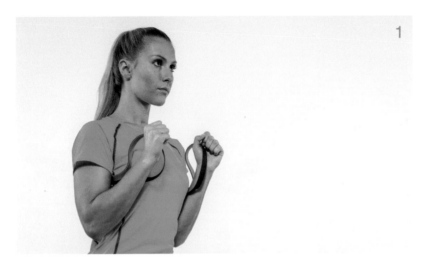

Photo 1: Place the band around your back just below the shoulder blades, and bring your arms to the front of the body. Hold it with both hands in front of the chest by placing a loop around each thumb as shown in the photo.

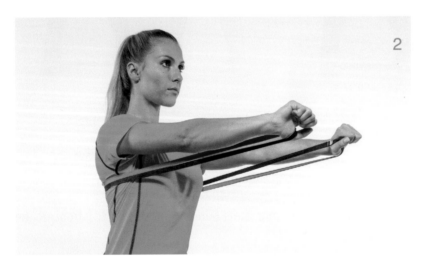

Photo 2: Now press your arms forward, either both at the same time or alternate, until they are fully extended. Keep repeating this motion sequence, slowly and steadily.

Resistance band pushups ✳✳✳

Shoulders, chest, triceps, abdominals

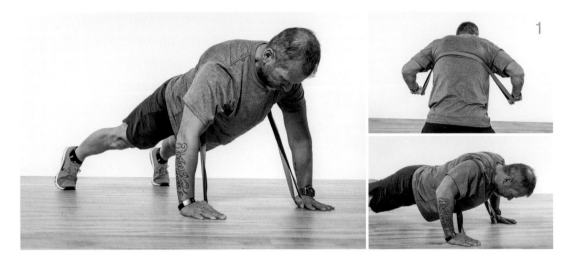

Photo 1: Like the previous "standing chest press" exercise, place the band around your back at chest level and hold it with both hands at the front of the body. Now get into classic pushup position.

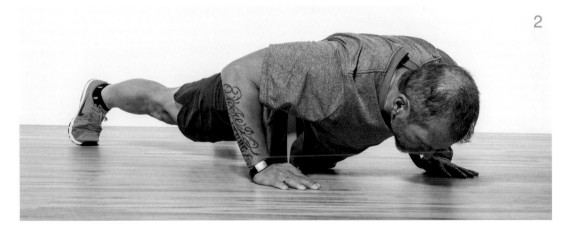

Photo 2: Perform pushups with the resistance of the band. The band's resistance makes this form of pushup more difficult than the traditional version..

Please note: make sure your abdominal muscles are engaged during all of the exercises.

Reclined chest press ✳✳

Shoulders, chest, triceps

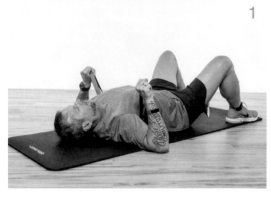

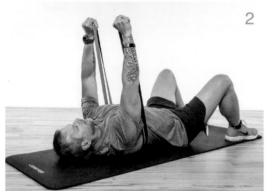

Photo 1: As with the two previous exercises, begin by placing the band across your back at chest level. Next, lie on your back on the floor, rest your elbows at your sides and hold both ends of the band in your hands. Bend your knees and plant your feet on the floor.

Photo 2: Now use your chest muscles to press the band upward until your arms are fully extended. The rest of the body remains still. Return your arms to the starting position. Keep repeating this motion sequence.

Alternative version:

Photo 3: Cross your arms as you press the band upward. By doing so, you will work the chest muscles even more.

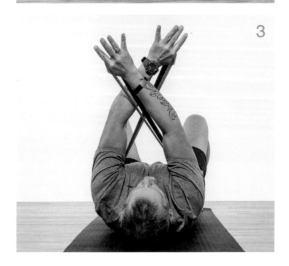

Bicep curls ✳✳

Biceps

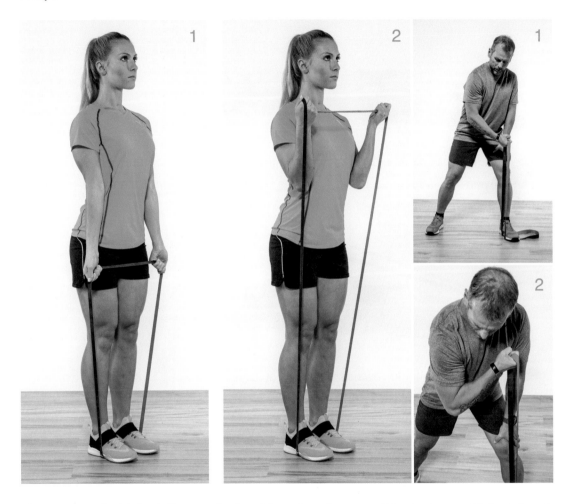

Photo 1: Stand with both feet on the band in a closed stance. Grip the band with both hands as shown in the photo. Let your arms hang loosely at the front of the body.

Photo 2: Now alternate bending and straightening your elbows. All the effort originates in the biceps. Make sure you have a steady and firm stance and engage your abdominal muscles during this exercise.

You can also perform this exercise with one arm, and then switch arms after a full set.

Reclined bicep curls ✳✳

Biceps

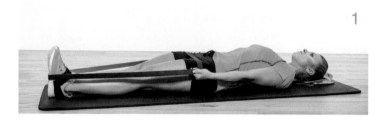

Photo 1: Lie on your back and extend your legs on the floor. Place the band around the bottom of your feet and add tension. Hold the band with both hands alongside your body with extended arms as shown in the photo.

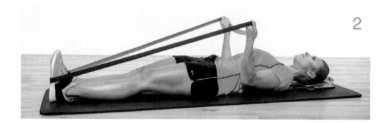

Photo 2: Now pull the band towards your chin by using your bicep muscles. Make sure the motion is clean and controlled. Other than your arms, your body should not move at all.

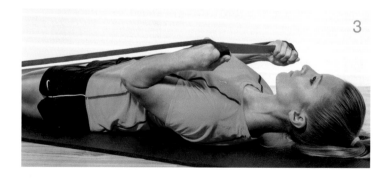

Photo 3: If you are strong enough, in the final position your hands may almost be at shoulder level. But you can also use a smaller range of motion as appropriate (see Photo 2).

Triceps press ✳✳✳

Triceps, shoulders

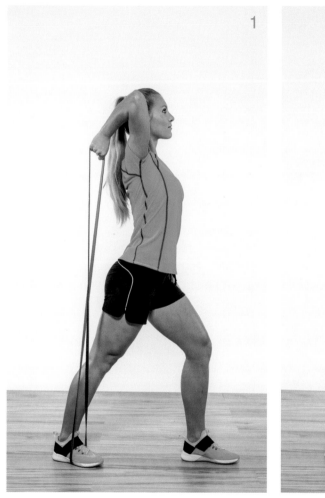
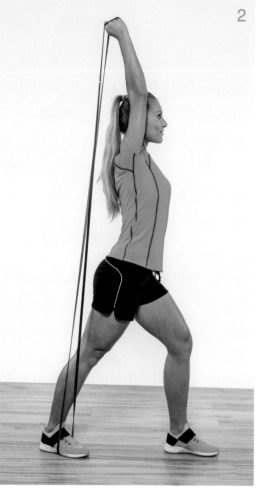

Photo 1: Stand with one foot on the band (right arm, right foot; left arm, left foot) and grip the band with both hands behind your head. In this position your elbows are bent. Make sure your stance is stable and your core muscles are engaged.

Photo 2: From this position, extend the arms up until they are all the way overhead. Perform this motion slowly, controlled, and strictly with the arms. The rest of the body should not move. Keep straightening and bending your elbows.

Boxing *

Shoulders, chest, triceps

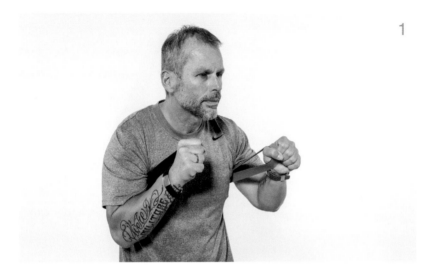

1

Photo 1: Place the band around your back at chest level and grip the ends with both hands. Close your hands into fists.

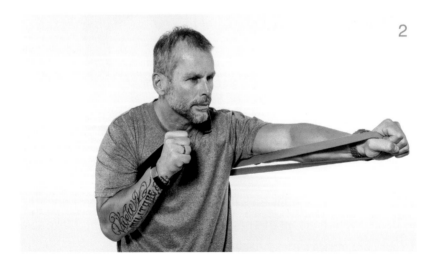

2

Photo 2: Now alternate extending your arms in front of your chest, like shadowboxing. You can alternate between your right and left arm or do multiple repetitions with one arm, and then switch.

Single-arm bent-over row ✳✳

Shoulders, back

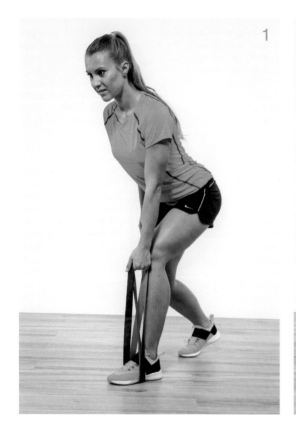 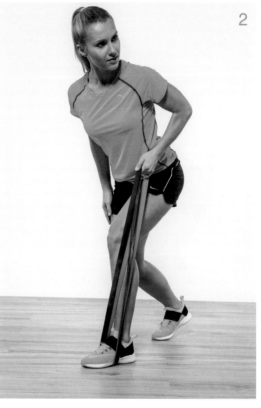

Photo 1: Double up on the band by folding it in half. Place one foot in the loop to hold down the band on the floor (see photo). Slightly bend your upper body forward while keeping your back straight. Step into a lunge and slightly bend your knees.

Photo 2: Now pull the elbow up as high as you can as close to the body as possible. Your leg position should not change. You can twist your upper body slightly to the side. As always, make sure your motion is slow and controlled.

Double-arm bent-over row ✳ ✳

Shoulders, back, thighs

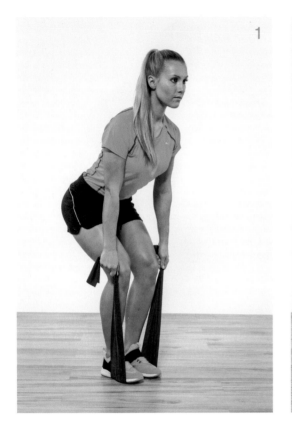
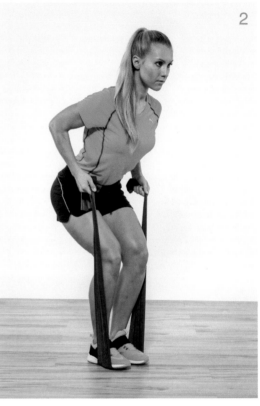

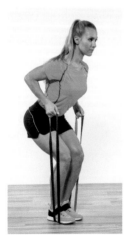

Photo 1: This exercise is similar to the previous one. You again hold the band down on the floor with your feet, slightly bend forward with your upper body, keep the back straight and slightly bend your knees. This time your feet should be parallel. Grip the band with both hands at knee level. Maintain extreme body tension.

Photo 2: The motion is similar to the previous exercise. This time, pull both elbows upward as far as you can, keeping the arms close to the body. Your hands are approximately at hip level.

You can do this as well as the other exercises with any level band appropriate for your fitness level.

Seated row *

Back, arms, shoulders

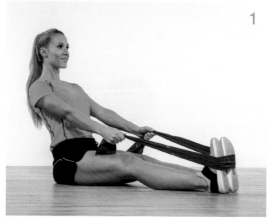

Photo 1: Sit on the floor with a straight back and your legs extended in front of you. Place the band around the bottom of your feet and grip the ends with both hands, arms fully extended.

Photo 2: Now pull the band towards you until your upper arms are at a 90-degree angle to your lower arms. The motion should be slow and controlled, using only the arms, and not moving the rest of the body.

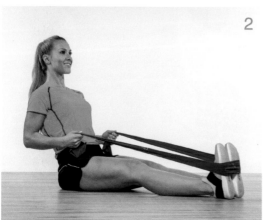

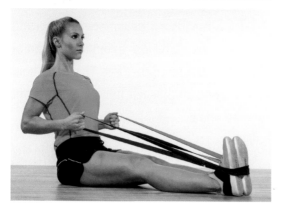

By using the highest level of resistance band, you can increase the resistance, which greatly increases the degree of difficulty.

Seated cross-band row ✳✳

Back, shoulders, arms

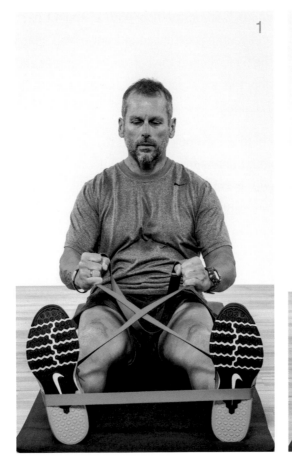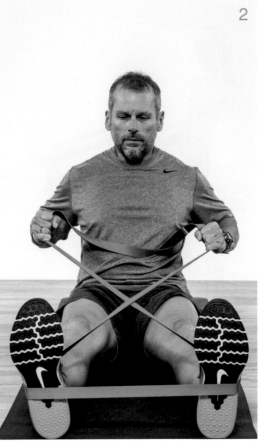

Photo 1: This exercise is also similar to the previous one but adds a little variety. The starting position will be the same. Sit on the floor with your back straight and legs extended in front of you (shoulder-width apart). The band is placed across the bottom of the feet. This time, hold the band crosswise, meaning the right hand grips the left end and the left hand grips the right end. Arms should be held at an approximate 90-degree angle.

Photo 2: Now pull the band towards you by moving your elbows as far back as possible. In the final position, your hands will be at about chest level. As always, make sure to maintain good body tension, especially in the trunk.

Overhead arm extension ✳✳

Back, shoulders, chest

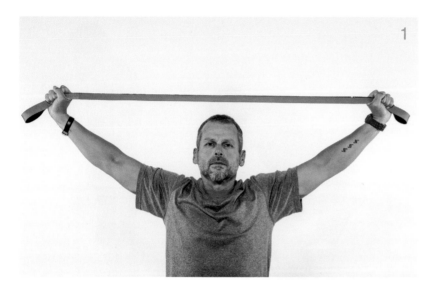

Photo 1: Stand upright and hold the band above your head as shown in the photo. Make sure the band is taut.

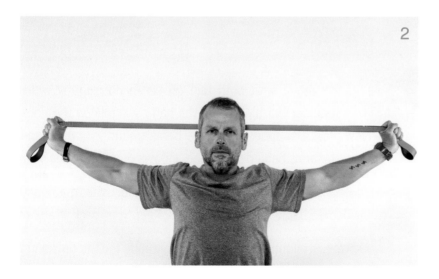

Photo 2: Now increase the tension in the band by lowering your arms slightly so that the band is behind your head.

Good mornings ✳✳

Lower back, legs

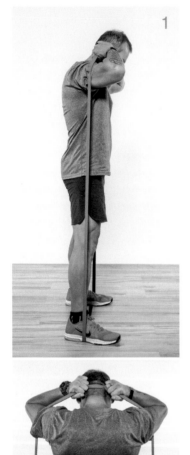

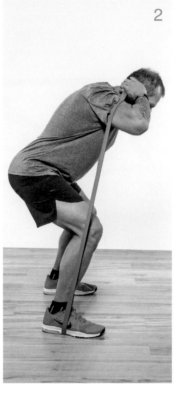

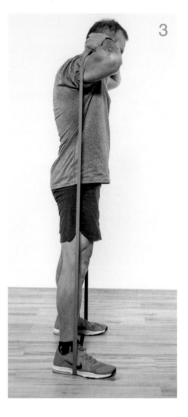

Photo 1: Stand with both feet on the band (slightly wider than shoulder-width), holding the band securely on the floor. Now place the upper end of the band around your nape and cross the arms behind your head, elbows pointing to the side.

Photo 2: Now bend your knees so your thighs are at a nearly 90-degree angle to your lower legs. Keep your back straight.

Photo 3: Straighten your body, maintaining muscle tension in your entire trunk. Keep repeating this motion sequence.

Squats ✳✳

Legs, core muscles

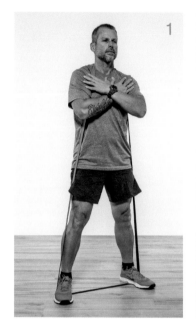 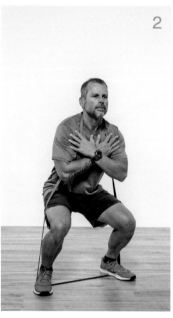 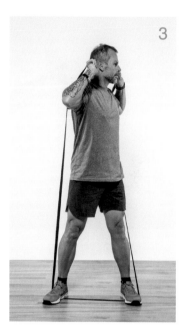

Photo 1: The starting position is similar to the previous exercise. You are again standing on the band with both feet, holding the band securely on the floor. Your legs are slightly more than shoulder-width apart. Place the upper end of the band around your nape. Stand upright and cross your arms in front of your chest.

Photo 2: Now do a classic squat by squatting down with a straight back. Keep your arms crossed in front of the chest. Next straighten up. Make sure to maintain muscle tension in your entire core during this exercise.

Alternative:

Photo 3: Add a rotating movement by alternately twisting to the left and right as you straighten up. This increases the intensity in abdominals and lower back.

If having the band across the nape feels unpleasant, you can hold onto it during the exercise instead of crossing your arms in front of your chest.

Leg press ✳✳

Legs, abdominals, lower back

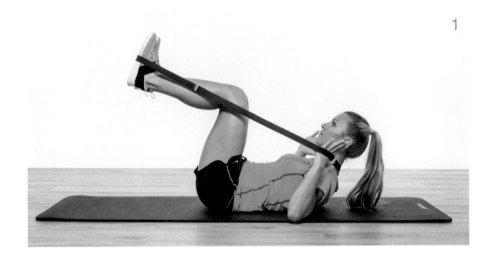

1

Photo 1: Lie on your back on the floor, raise your legs and bend your knees. Next, raise your upper body a couple inches off of the floor. Place one end of the band around the bottom of your feet and the other end around your neck. Use your hands to push the band slightly out to the sides and your elbows propped on the floor.

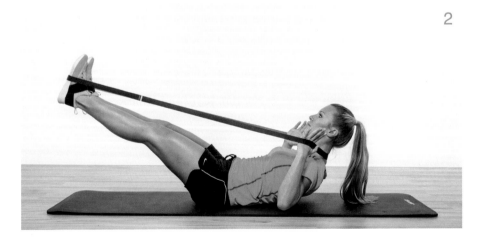

2

Photo 2: Now press your feet forward against the band's resistance, using your thigh muscles, until your legs are fully extended. The position of the upper body should not change.

Leg extension ✳✳

Abdominals, iliopsoas muscles, calves

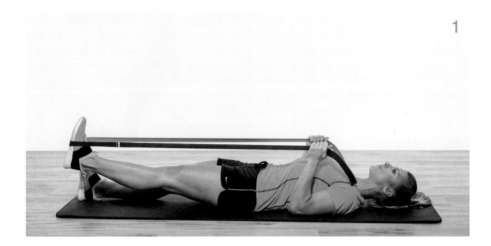

Photo 1: Begin by lying on your back on the floor with your legs extended. Place the upper end of the band around your neck and the lower end around the bottom of the left foot. Grip the band with your hands at chest level as shown in the photo. Raise the left leg a couple inches off of the floor.

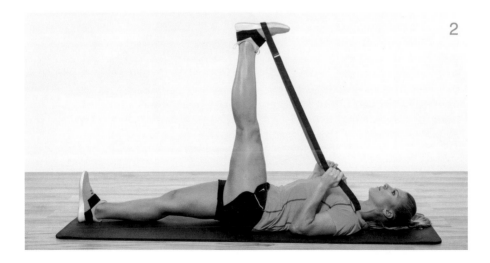

Photo 2: Now pull the fully extended leg up until it is in a vertical position and at a right angle to the floor. Keep repeating this motion sequence. Switch legs after completing a full set.

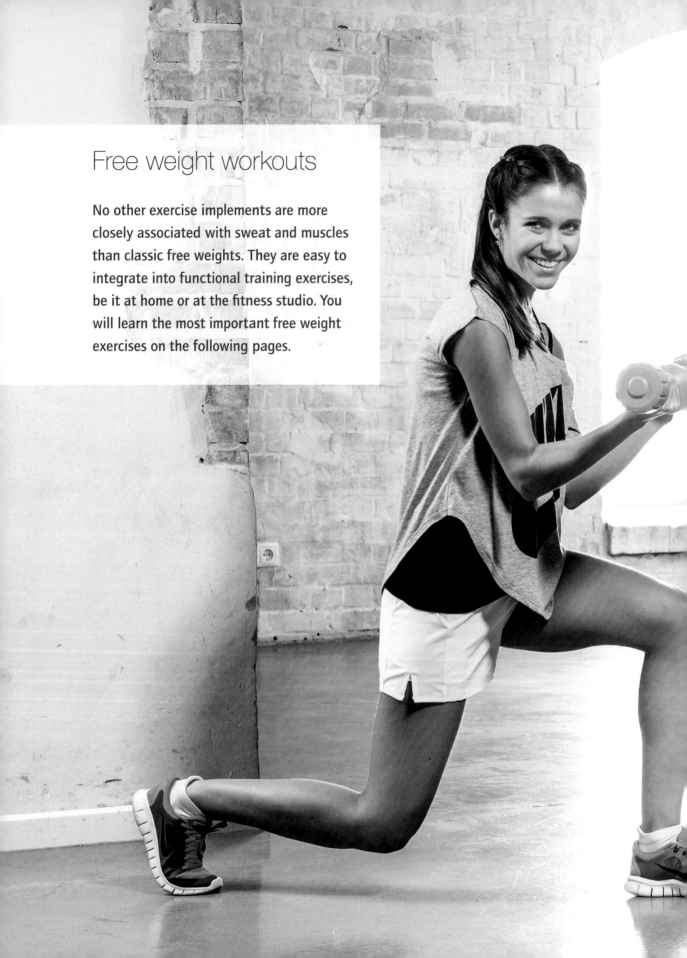

Free weight workouts

No other exercise implements are more closely associated with sweat and muscles than classic free weights. They are easy to integrate into functional training exercises, be it at home or at the fitness studio. You will learn the most important free weight exercises on the following pages.

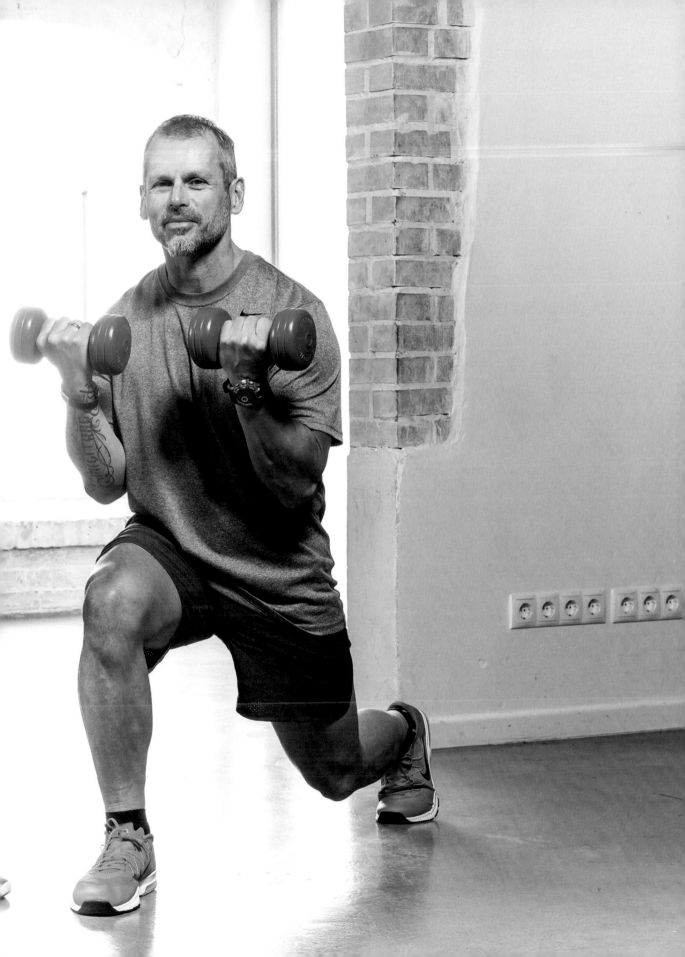

Hammer curls ✳

Biceps

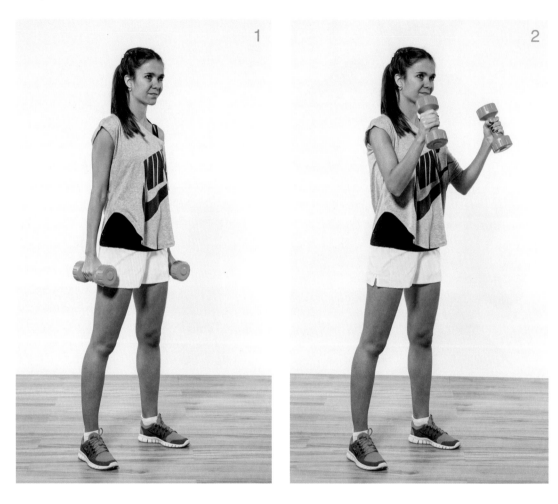

Photo 1: Stand in an upright position with your feet slightly more than shoulder-width apart. The arms should hang loosely at your sides and you will hold the weights like a hammer.

Photo 2: Now raise the weights by using your biceps muscles. In the final position, the weights are approximately at shoulder level. You should not rotate your hands, hence the name hammer curls. Try to keep your upper arms still and close to your body. Return the weights to the starting position.

Biceps curls ✻

Biceps

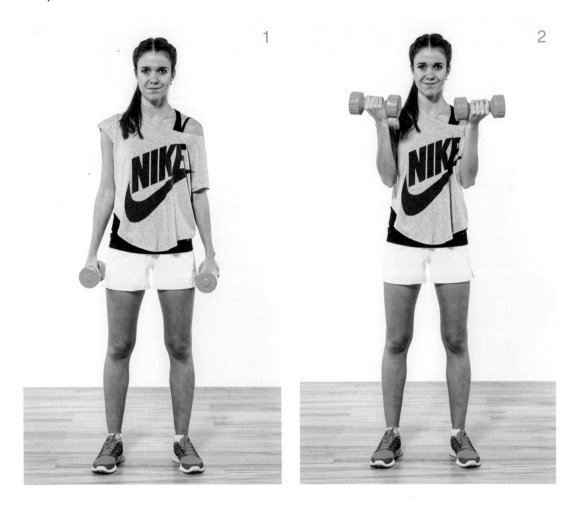

Photo 1, Photo 2: The starting position is the same as the exercise "hammer curls." The motion sequence is also similar. This time, you rotate your forearms so that the backs of the hands point to the outside in the final position. This works the biceps more intensively than the hammer curls.

Alternative:
You can do hammer or bicep curls with one arm at a time.

Reclined chest press ✳✳

Chest, shoulders, triceps

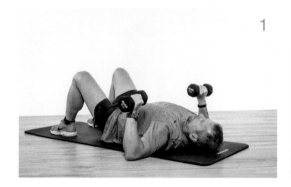
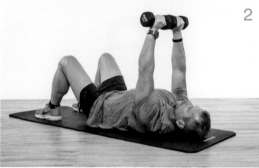

Photo 1: Classic bench-press – but without the bench. Lie on your back with knees bent and feet planted. The upper arms are at a right angle to the forearms and the elbows point to the side. Hold the weights over the chest with the back of your hands facing you.

Photo 2: From this position, press the weights up above the chest until the arms are fully extended. Then lower them back down.

A tip from Mike

Do you want to make the exercise more intense and work your deep muscles harder? Then go back to the stability ball. Lie on your back on the ball and steady yourself with your feet against the floor. Maintain maximum muscle tension in the trunk. Now press the weights upward, alternating arms.

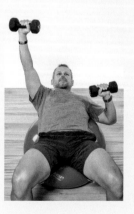
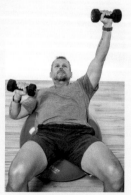

Chest flys on the stability ball ✳✳

Chest, shoulders

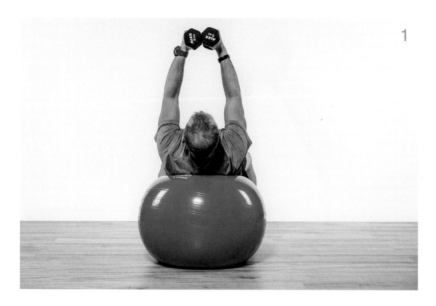

Photo 1: Aou will need a stability ball for this exercise. Lie on your back on the ball with your knees bent and your feet planted on the floor. Slightly raise your upper body and hips and hold the weights overhead with your arms extended.

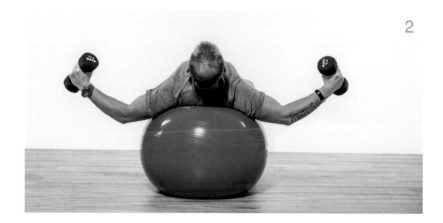

Photo 2: Now lower the arms to your sides in a semi-circular motion. In the final position, the weights should be at about shoulder level. Next, return the arms to the starting position.

Reclined triceps press ✳

Triceps

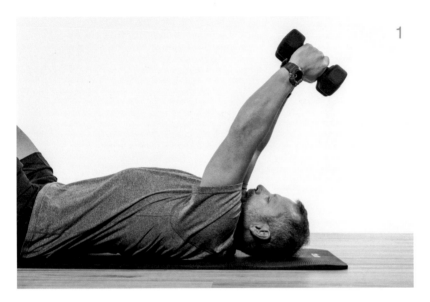

Photo 1: Lie on your back on the floor with knees bent and feet planted on the floor. Hold the weights in your hands with your arms extended overhead and the backs of your hands pointing to the outside.

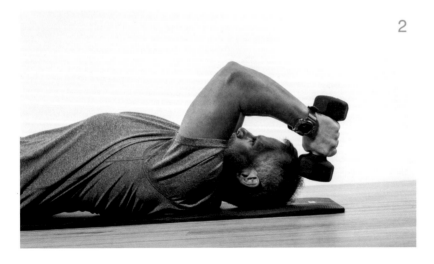

Photo 2: Slowly bend and straighten the arms as shown in the photos.

Reclined pullover with triceps extension ✳✳✳

Triceps, chest, back

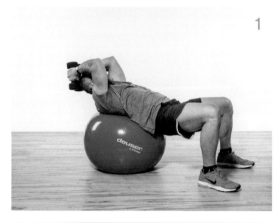

1

Photo 1: Here we use the stability ball again. Lie on your back on the ball and steady yourself with your legs. Hold the weights behind your head in a hammer grip with elbows bent.

Photo 2: Fully extend the arms.

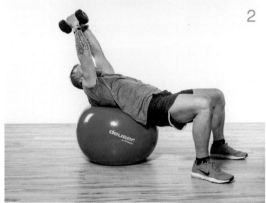

2

Photo 3: Move them as far back as you can to work both the chest and back muscles. Then raise the extended arms again and bend the elbows to return to the starting position.

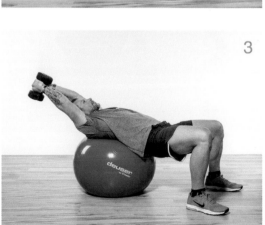

3

Standing triceps kickbacks ✳

Triceps, shoulders

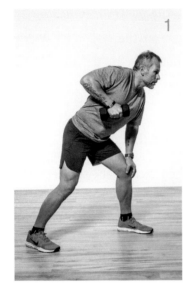 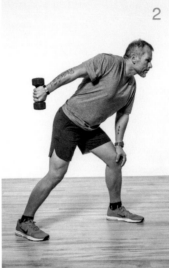

Photo 1: Step into a lunge and brace yourself with your left arm on your right knee. Hold the weight in your right hand in a hammer grip with the elbow bent.

Photo 2: Now straighten the arm by pressing the forearm back to achieve optimal muscle tension in the triceps. Briefly hold this position and then bend the elbow again.

A tip from Mike

Want a little variety? Grab the stability ball and support yourself on it. The bent-over posture works the back muscles more.

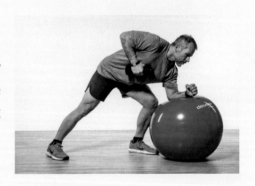

Static lunge with curls **

All of the thigh muscles, biceps, core

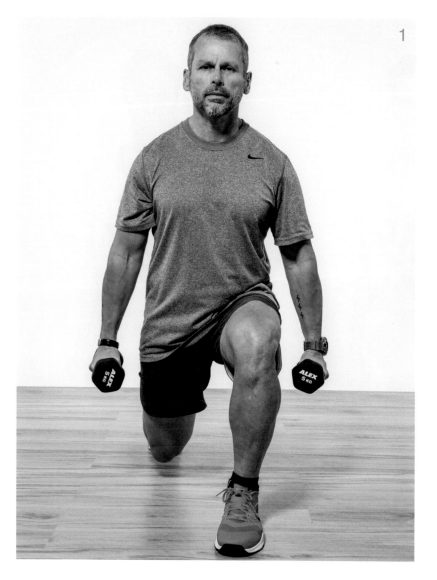

Photo 1: Step into a classic lunge. Hold this position during the entire exercise. Now do bicep curls, either with both or alternating arms (see first exercise). Switch legs after one set. Instead of bicep curls, you can also do hammer curls.

Lunge with weights *

All thigh muscles

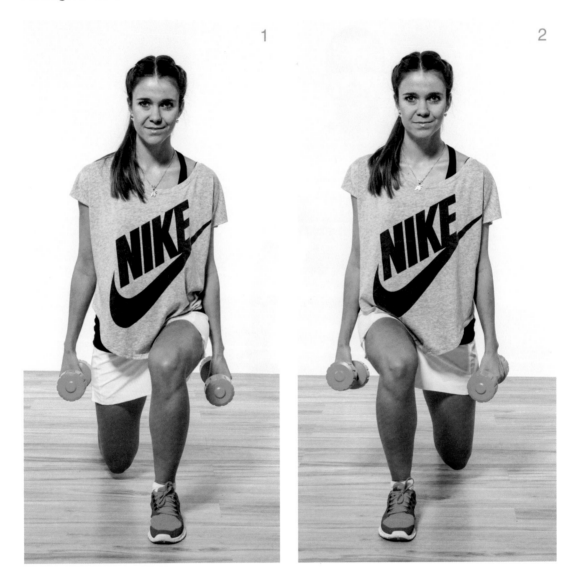

1

2

Photo 1, Photo 2: You are already familiar with the lunge from the previous exercises. But this time you should hold weights in your hands, which helps to increase the intensity. Make sure your core muscles are engaged.

Squats with weights ✳ ✳

All thigh muscles, gluteals

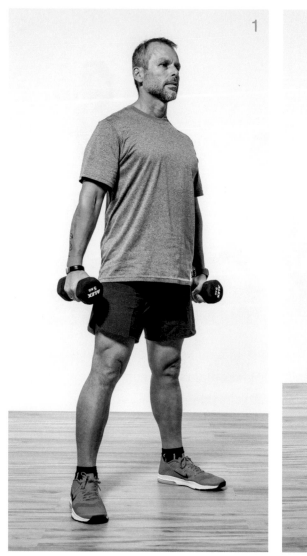 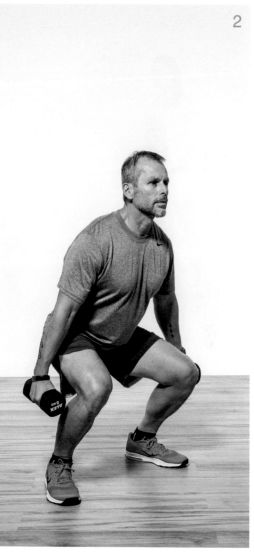

Photo 1, Photo 2: Stand upright with your feet slightly more than shoulder-width apart. Hold the weights in a hammer grip with your arms extended at your sides. Now lower your bottom by engaging your thigh muscles until your thighs are at an approximate 90-degree angle to your lower legs. Slowly push back up from this position.

Squat with shoulder press ✳✳✳

All thigh muscles, gluteals, core, shoulders

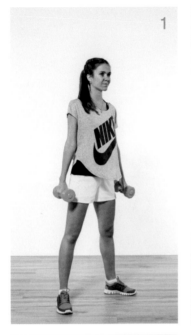

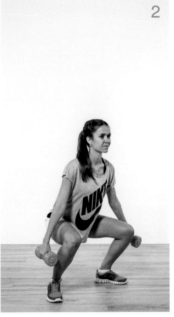

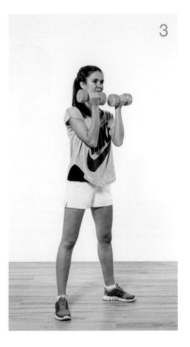

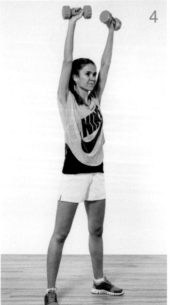

Photo 1: This exercise requires lots of coordination. Stand upright and hold the weights in a hammer grip with your arms extended at your sides.

Photo 2: As with the previous exercise, move into a squat.

Photo 3: Push yourself back up into an upright position while simultaneously bending the elbows so that the weights are at chin level.

Photo 4: Slowly press the weights overhead while engaging your abdominal muscles. Next reverse the motion sequence and repeat the exercise.

Dumbbell swing ✳✳✳

All thigh muscles, core, shoulders

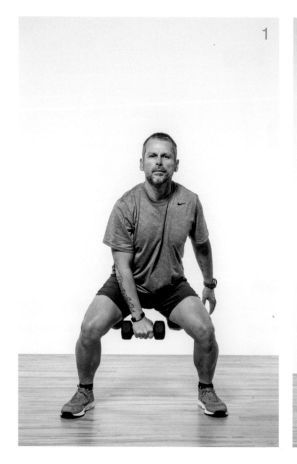 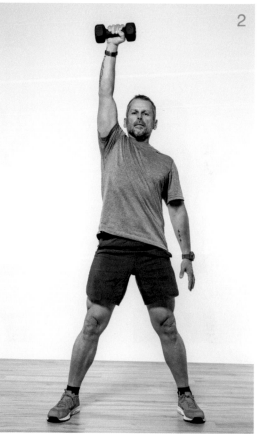

Photo 1: Position your feet slightly more than shoulder-width apart. Hold the weight between your knees with the arm fully extended, the back of the hand facing away from you. Make sure your back is straight!

Photo 2: Vigorously push up out of this position with your knees, while simultaneously jerking the weight overhead with the extended arm.

Please note:

this exercise is only suitable for experienced exercisers. People with shoulder or back problems should not try to do this exercise..

Dumbbell shoulder press ✳✳

Shoulders

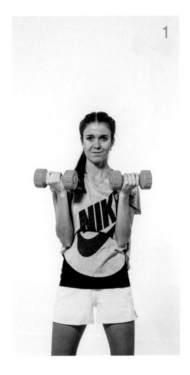
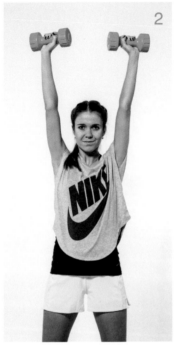

Photo 1: Assume a stable stance. Hold the weights at shoulder level with your elbows bent and the backs of your hands facing outward.

Photo 2: From this position, press the weights as far overhead as you can until your arms are fully extended. During this motion, rotate your arms 180 degrees. The backs of your hands will now face backwards. Now slowly return the arms to the starting position.

A tip from Mike

Performing this exercise while sitting on a stability ball is much easier on the back.

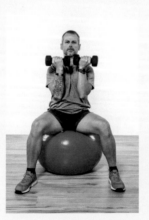
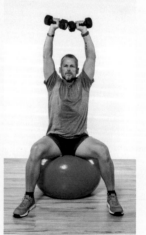

Upright row **

Shoulders, trapezius

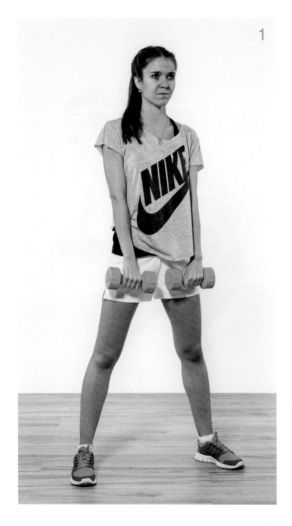 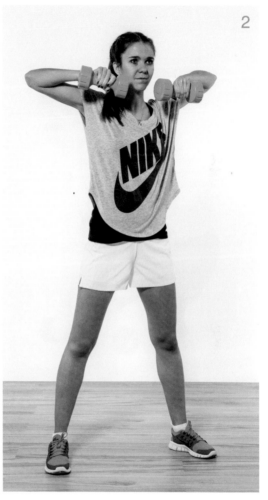

Photo 1: Assume a stable stance with your feet slightly more than shoulder-width apart. Hold the weights at the front of the body with arms extended, the backs of your hands facing away from you.

Photo 2: Now pull the weights up until your upper arms and shoulders form a straight line. Elbows should be pointing to the outside. Next, return to the starting position, making sure your movements are slow and controlled.

Bent-over row ✳✳

Latissimus dorsi, shoulders

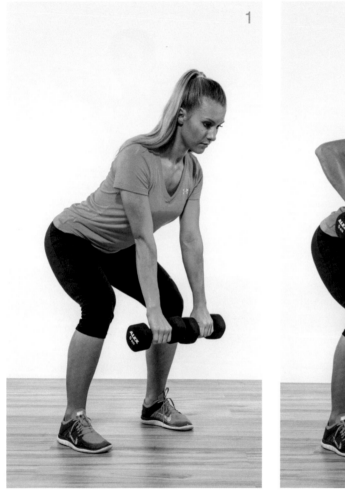 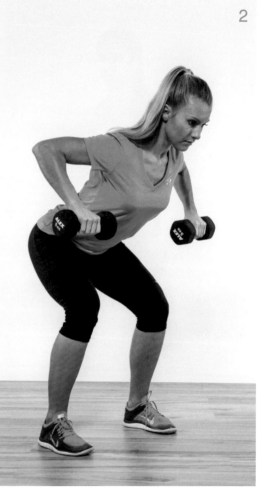

Photo 1: Stand with your feet shoulder-width apart and knees bent as shown in the photo. Keep your back straight. Hold the weights slightly below knee level with the arms extended. The backs of the hands should face forward.

Photo 2: Slowly and steadily, pull both arms backwards leading with the elbows, until the upper arms are at a right angle to the forearms. Briefly hold this position and then return to the starting position.

Bent-over lateral raises ✳✳

Shoulders, thigh muscles

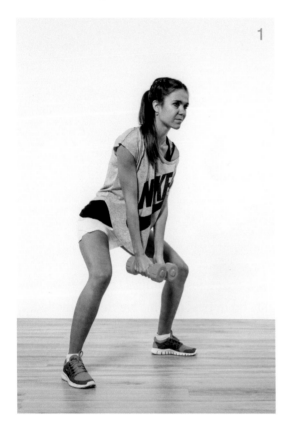 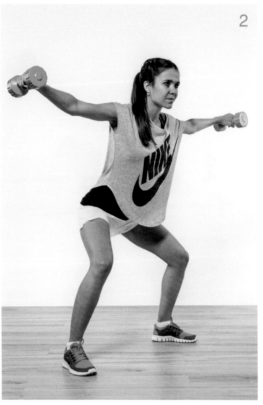

Photo 1: Place your feet wider than shoulder-width apart. Bend your knees so that you are in a comfortable position.

Please note: you can also perform this exercise in an upright position, or bend the knees even more than shown in the photo.

Important: keep your back straight. Hold the weights between your knees in a hammer grip with extended arms.

Photo 2: Now raise your arms sideways until the weights are approximately at shoulder level. The upper body should not move during this motion.

Crunches with free weights ✳✳

Abdominals, lower back, shoulders, chest

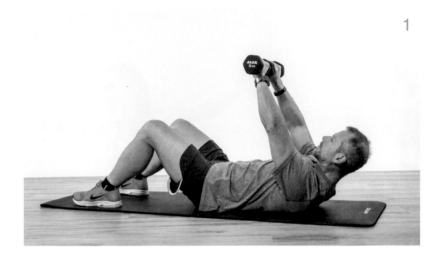

1

Photo 1: Lie on your back on the floor, bend your knees and rest your heels on the floor. Now raise your upper body slightly and press the weights up until your arms are fully extended.

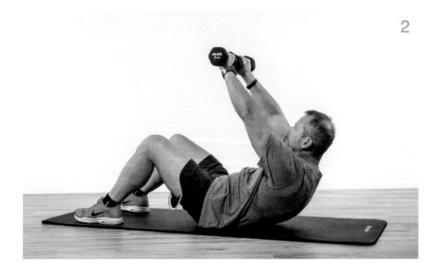

2

Photo 2: From this position, lift your trunk as high as possible, working only the abdominal muscles. Then lower yourself back down to the starting position. The arms should not move at all during this exercise.

Pushup to row ✳✳✳

Whole-body exercise

1

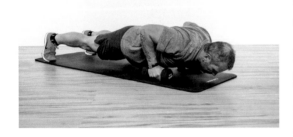

Photo 1: This is a killer exercise to close this chapter. Get into classic pushup position, holding the weights in a hammer grip, and lower your body until the tip of your nose almost touches the floor.

Photo 2: Next push yourself back up until your arms are fully extended.

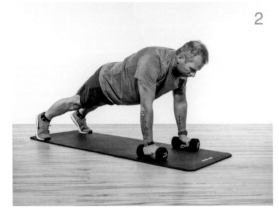

2

Photo 3: Then pull one elbow back up as far as you can. The elbow should point to the ceiling. Return to the starting position, repeat the pushup, and then perform the rowing motion with the other arm.

3

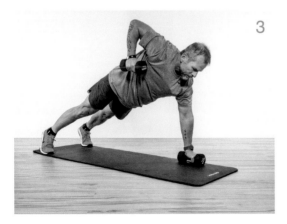

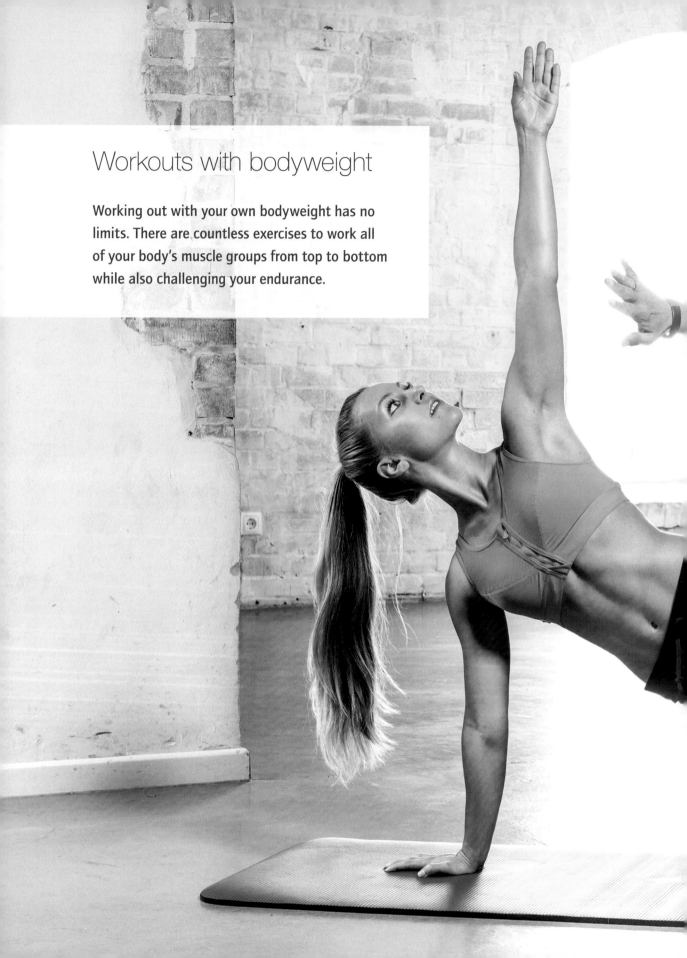

Workouts with bodyweight

Working out with your own bodyweight has no limits. There are countless exercises to work all of your body's muscle groups from top to bottom while also challenging your endurance.

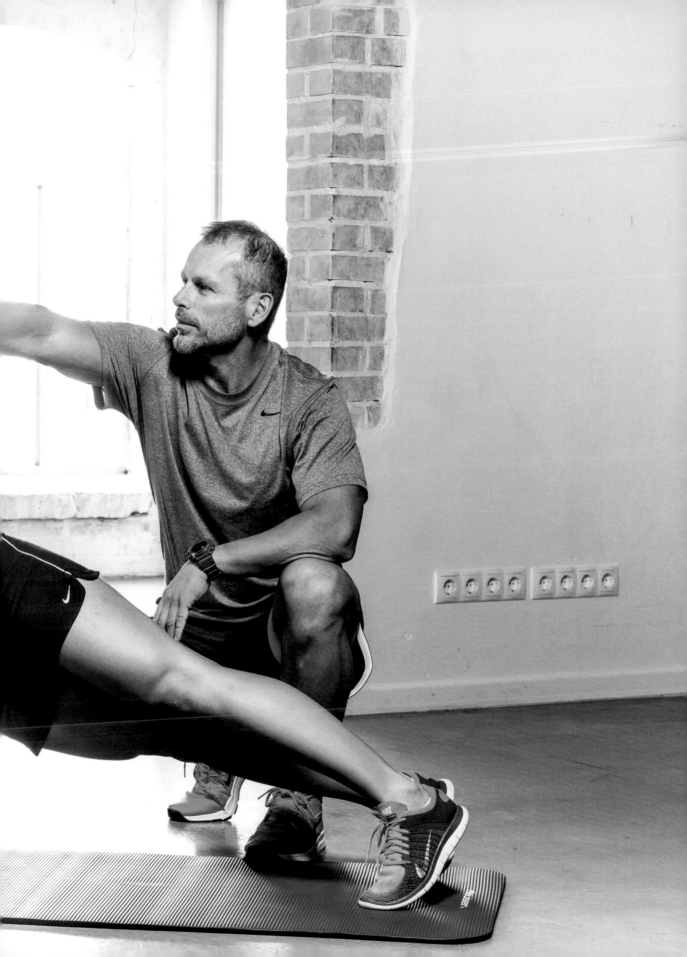

Strength and endurance

Hardly any other exercise will burn as much fat as endurance-oriented bodyweight workouts. With respect to endurance, the following exercises are extremely strenuous and effective.

Burpees

Whole-body exercise

1

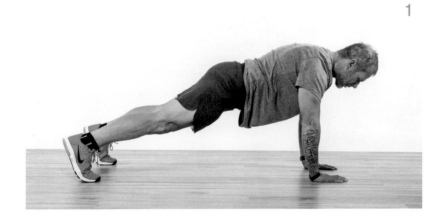

2

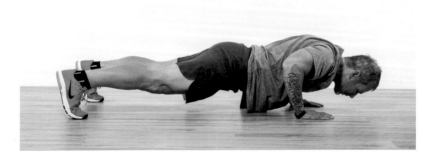

Photo 1, Photo 2: Begin in classic pushup position, bend the elbows and lower your body until the tip of your nose almost touches the floor.

3

4

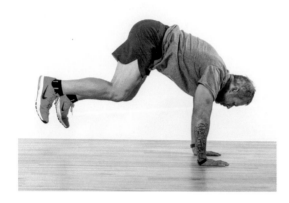
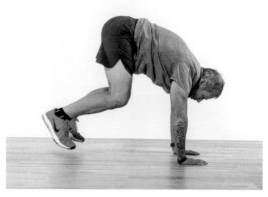

Photo 3, Photo 4: After pushing yourself back up into starting position, jump into a squat with both legs.

5

6

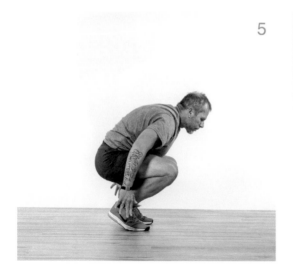
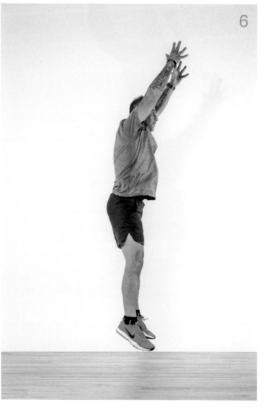

Photo 5, Photo 6: Take your hands off the floor and shift your bodyweight backwards. Then jump straight up into the air with legs extended, and arms overhead. Then immediately return to the pushup position and repeat the entire motion sequence.

High knees ✳✳

Legs, gluteals, core

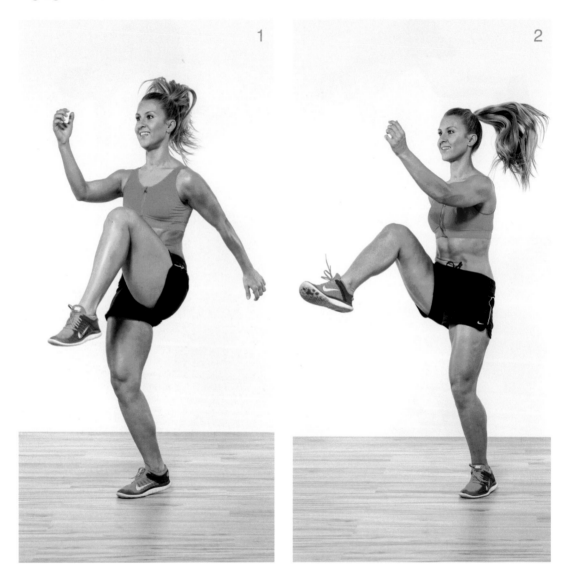

Photo 1, Photo 2: Begin in an upright position with your feet shoulder-width apart. Now pull your knees as close as possible to your chest, alternating between legs. The arms should simultaneously swing in the opposite direction.

Jumping jacks ✳✳

All leg muscles, gluteals, core, shoulders

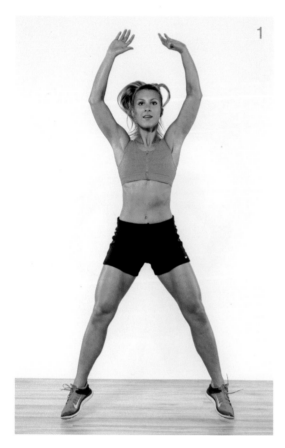

Photo 1: Begin by standing with your feet shoulder-width apart. The arms should hang loosely at your sides. Vigorously jump up and simultaneously swing your arms up overhead. At the same time, open your legs into a straddle in the air. Land softly into the starting position and immediately repeat the motion sequence.

A tip from Mike

Does this sound like a silly children's exercise to you? Think again! Jumping jacks are perfect for a warm-up exercise. This movement also gets your heart pumping. Try the following challenge: 5 x 50 repetitions with 10-50 second breaks in ascending order in-between sets. Strenuous enough?

Butt kicks ✳✳

Front of thighs, iliopsoas muscles, abdominals, lower back

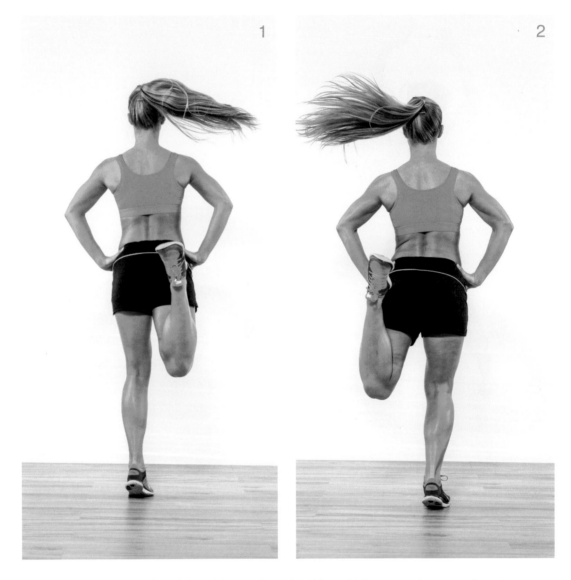

Photo 1, Photo 2: Stand upright with your feet shoulder-width apart. Place your hands on your hips. Now alternate vigorously, pulling your left and right heel towards your bottom. Make sure to perform this exercise as vigorously as possible, and you will feel that it will become quite strenuous after a while.

Mountain climbers ✳✳

Whole-body exercise

1

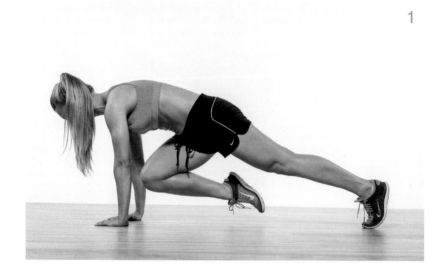

2

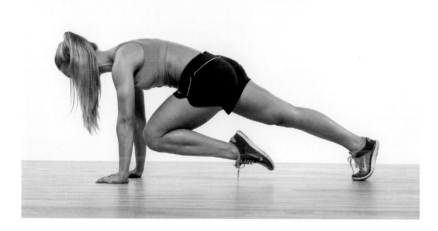

This is a classic bodyweight exercise and will also make you sweat after a while.

Photo 1, Photo 2: Get down on all fours. From this position, vigorously jump forward with one leg, alternating legs.

Shadowboxing ✳

Shoulders, arms, chest, abdominals, lower back

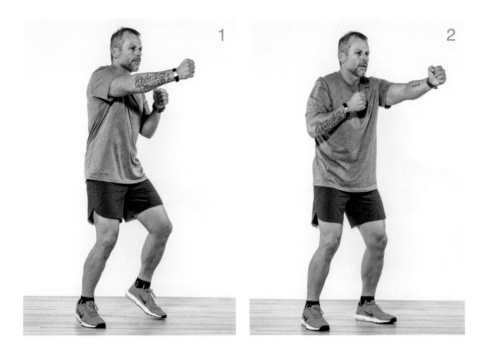

Photo 1, Photo 2: Imagine yourself standing in the ring like Rocky Balboa used to do, fighting the match of your life. However, instead of striking your opponent with your fists, your left and right hooks should only land in the air. At the same time, you bob and weave and stay in constant motion. You can intensify shadowboxing by punching faster or slower, moving more vigorously or slowly. It is also an ideal warm-up exercise..

A tip from Mike

All of these exercises that are particularly hugely effective for endurance training work very well with a Tabata-style approach (8 x 20 seconds with 10-second breaks in-between) as individual circuits. You can also look at the circuits at the back of the book.

Upper body

Muscular arms, broad shoulders, and a strong back are considered visual ideals, at least for men. However, women are now also increasingly focusing on building a fitter body. The following exercises will help you work your upper half.

Bicep curls ✳✳

Biceps

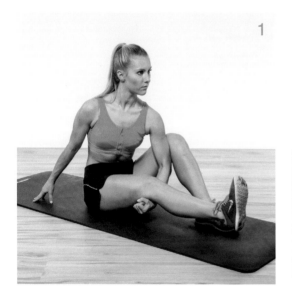 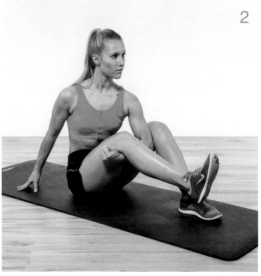

Photo 1: You can't work your biceps without weights? Nonsense! You can shape your upper arms just as effectively without implements. Place your left upper arm against the inside of your right thigh. Close your hand into a fist and slide it under the back of your right knee. Support yourself on the floor with your right hand.

Photo 2: Now use the strength of your biceps to pull your right leg towards your chest. Then guide it back to the starting position, again working against your leg's resistance. After completing one set, switch sides.

Dips ✳✳

Triceps, shoulders

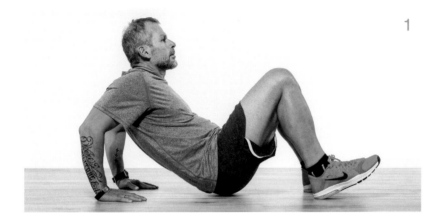

1

Photo 1: Begin in a seated position. Bend your knees and let your heels rest on the floor. Support yourself with your hands on the floor behind your back. The elbows should be slightly bent and fingertips pointing forward.

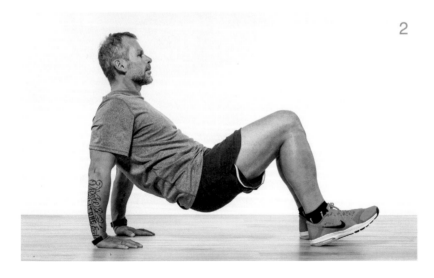

2

Photo 2: Now push yourself up until your arms are fully extended, using the strength of your triceps. Then return to the starting position.

Important: don't let your bottom touch the floor!

Triceps kickbacks ✳✳

Triceps, shoulders

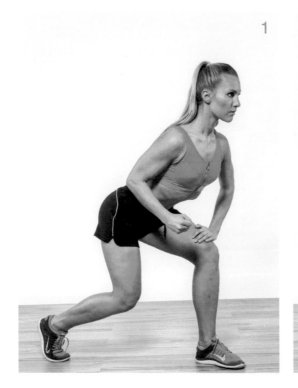
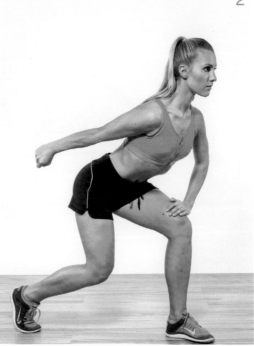

Photo 1: Step into a lunge position and support yourself with your left arm on your left knee. Lean forward slightly with your upper body, keeping your back straight. Bend the right elbow to a right angle with your upper arm remaining parallel to your trunk.

Photo 2: Now extend the forearm back, generating maximum tension in the triceps. Briefly hold this position and then bend the elbow again.

Harder version: hold an object in your hand to work the triceps even harder, for example a water bottle. After completing one set, switch arms.

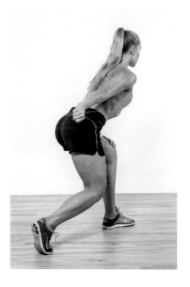

Classic pushups ✳✳✳

Whole-body exercise

1

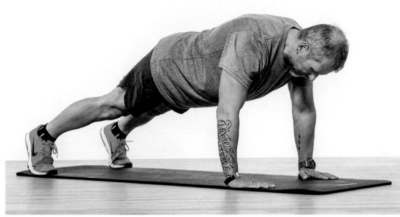

Photo 1: This is hands-down the classic bodyweight exercise. First, get into classic pushup position. Your hands and feet should remain shoulder-width apart.

2

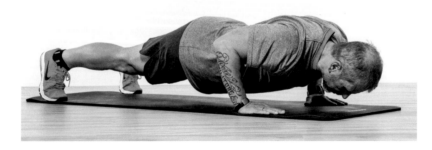

Photo 2: Now lower your body until the tip of your nose almost touches the floor, then push yourself back up until your arms are fully extended.

More variations

Triangle pushups ✳✳✳

Emphasis on: triceps, chest
Other muscles: shoulders, abdominals, lower back

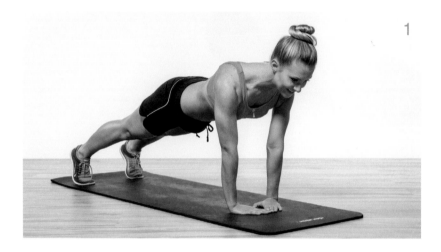

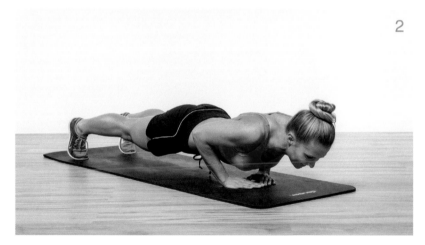

Photo 1, Photo 2: **Heads up! This is a brutal exercise. Position your hands close enough together so that your thumbs and forefingers touch. The rest of the motion sequence should not change. This version primarily works the triceps.**

Wide grip pushups ✳✳✳

Emphasis on: chest, latissimus dorsi
Other muscles: shoulders, triceps, abdominals

1

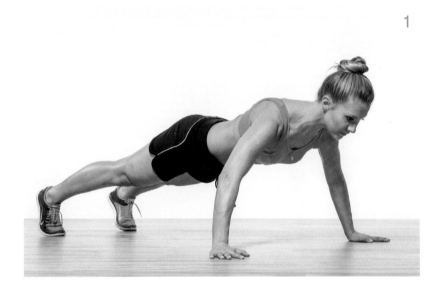

2

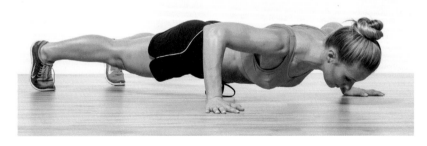

Photo 1, Photo 2: For this version of the pushup, place your hands much farther apart. This will result in working the muscles in the upper back.

Side-to-side pushups ✳✳✳

Emphasis on: chest, shoulders
Other muscles: triceps, abdominals, lower back

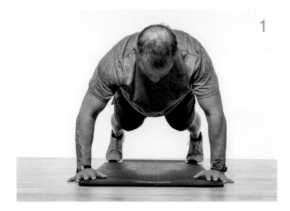

1

Photo 1: Get in classic pushup position with your hands slightly more than shoulder-width apart.

Photo 2, Photo 3: Now lower your upper body towards your left hand. Then push yourself back up to the starting position with a rolling motion of the upper body. Then lower down towards your right hand.

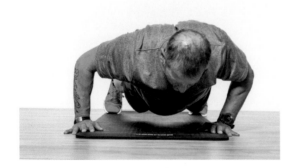

2

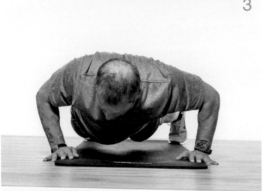

3

Pushups with core rotation ✳✳

Emphasis in: abdominals, lower back (core)
Other muscles: shoulders, triceps

1

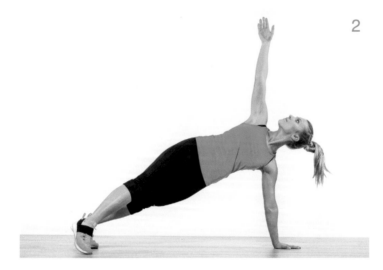

Photo 1: Get into classic pushup position. Hands should be placed below shoulders with your arms held close to the body. Now lower your body until the tip of your nose almost touches the floor.

2

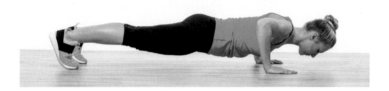

Photo 2: Push yourself back up until your arms are extended, and rotate to one side to open up your upper body. One arm is extended to the ceiling as shown in the photo. Your eyes track the arm motion. Then return to pushup position, push yourself up again and rotate the upper body to the other side.

Plank to pushup ✳✳

Emphasis on: chest, shoulders
Other muscles: abdominals, lower back, triceps

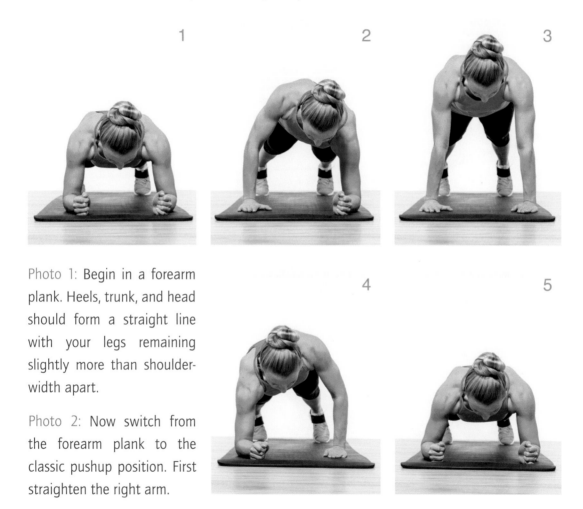

Photo 1: Begin in a forearm plank. Heels, trunk, and head should form a straight line with your legs remaining slightly more than shoulder-width apart.

Photo 2: Now switch from the forearm plank to the classic pushup position. First straighten the right arm.

Photo 3: And then the left arm.

Photo 4: Then immediately return to the forearm plank. First with the right arm.

Photo 5: And then with the left arm.

Floor row ✳✳

Latissimus dorsi, abdominals

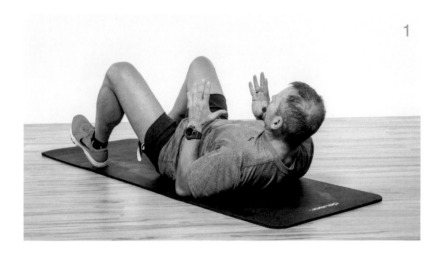

1

Photo 1: Lie on your back on the floor. Bend your knees and let your heels rest on the floor. Slightly raise your shoulders and create muscle tension. As shown in the photo, prop yourself up on your elbows, keeping them close to your body.

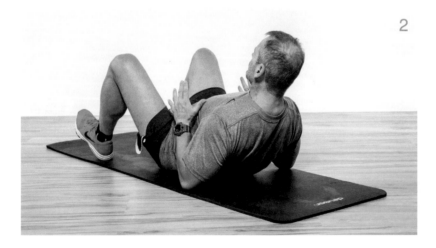

2

Photo 2: Now press your elbows into the floor and lift your upper body a little higher. Hold this position for 1-2 seconds, and lower back down.

Important: do not rest your back on the floor during the entire exercise.

Dynamic bridge ✳✳

Core, shoulders, chest, calves

1

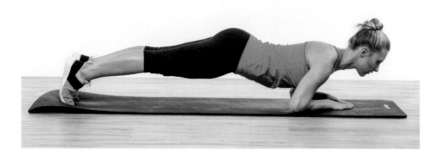

Photo 1: Begin in a forearm plank. Heels, upper body, and head should form a nearly straight line.

2

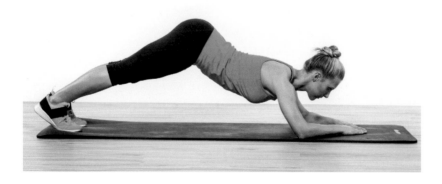

Photo 2: Now push your trunk and bottom upward as far as you can so that your body forms a bridge. The arm position should not change. Hold this position for 1-2 seconds, and lower back down into the starting position.

Shoulder rolls ✳

Shoulders upper back

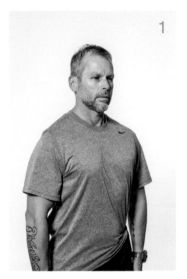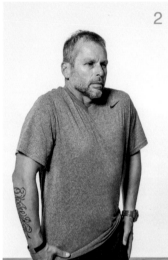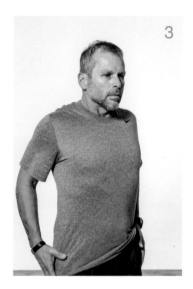

Photo 1: Stand with your feet shoulder-width apart, arms touching your sides. Make sure your abdominals and low-back muscles are engaged.

Photo 2, Photo 3: Now alternate rolling your shoulders forward and back in circles.

Lateral raises ✳

Shoulders

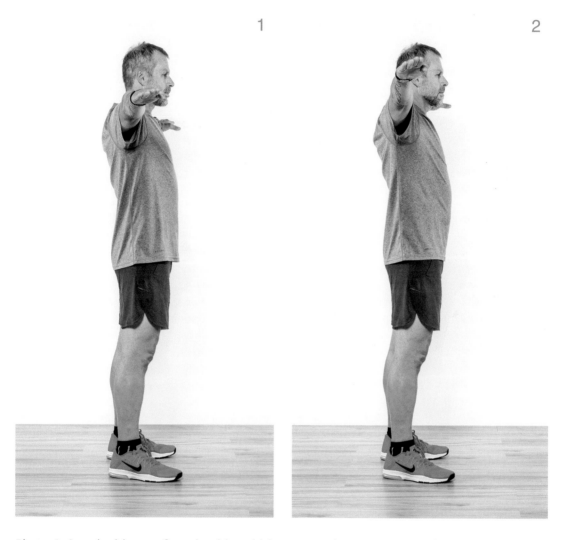

Photo 1: Stand with your feet shoulder-width apart. Raise your arms to the sides to shoulder level with your palms facing the floor.

Photo 2: Now raise your arms a few more inches. In the final position, they should be at approximately ear level. Then immediately lower them again. Be sure to maintain body tension during the entire exercise.

Lateral arm extension ✳

Shoulders

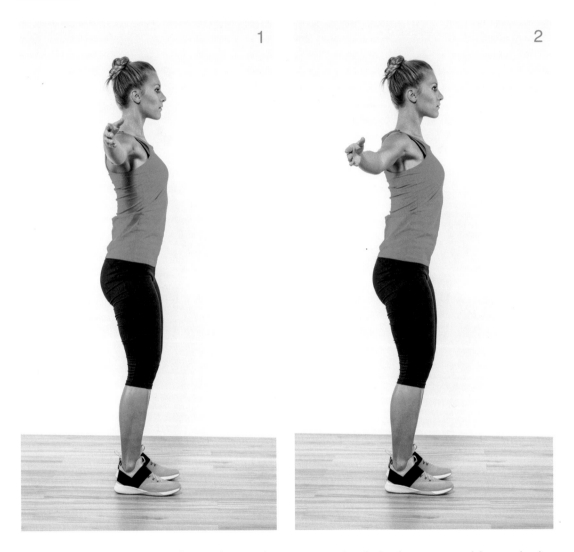

Photo 1: This exercise is similar to the previous one. You begin in the same position and raise your arms to shoulder level. However, this time the palms will face forward.

Photo 2: Now push your extended arms as far back as possible and then return them to the starting position. Make sure to only briefly move your arms back and forth and keep your core muscles engaged.

Bent-over lateral raises *

Shoulders, core

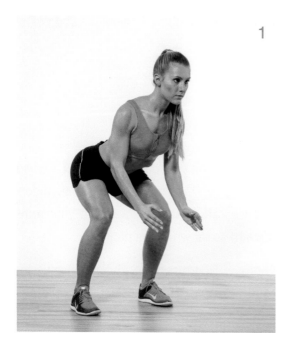
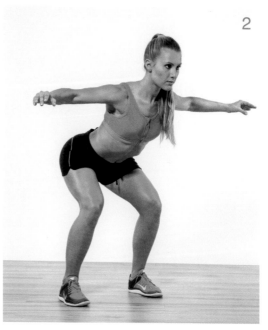

Photo 1: Place your feet slightly more than shoulder-width apart. Bend forward slightly with your upper body and then bend your knees. Extend your arms downward in front of the body. Maintain muscle tension in your hands.

Photo 2: Now pull your extended arms back until your hands are at shoulder level. Hold this position for about one second. Return to the starting position.

Important: be sure to maintain muscle tension in your trunk during this exercise.

A tip from Mike

You can easily make the last three exercises more difficult by holding weights or water bottles in each hand.

Belly and back

Who doesn't dream of having a six-pack, the ideal beach body? A strong back will also prevent back problems and postural defects. The following exercises will primarily work the abdominal muscles and back.

Dynamic sit-ups ✳ ✳

Abdominals, lower back

1

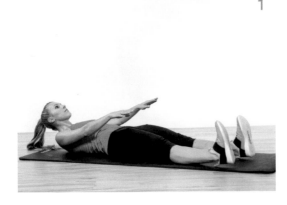

Photo 1: Lie on your back on the floor. Extend your legs and slightly raise your shoulders and legs off of the floor. Extend your arms forward as shown in the photo.

Photo 2: Now use your abdominal muscles to pull up to a seated position as upright as possible. As you do so, bend your knees and let your heels rest on the floor. Afterwards return to the starting position.

2

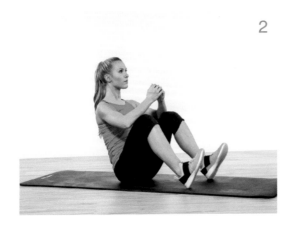

Swimmer ✳✳

Lower back, shoulders

1

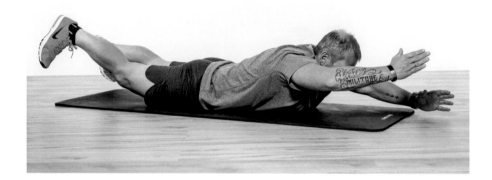

2

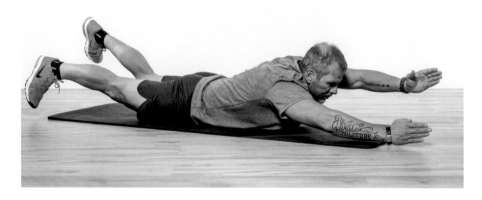

Photo 1, Photo 2: Lie on your stomach on the floor and extend your arms and legs, raising them a couple inches off of the floor. Then alternate between lifting one arm and one leg. Perform this exercise and alternate between sides. Maintain whole-body tension during the entire exercise.

Russian Twist ✳✳

Abdominals, lower back

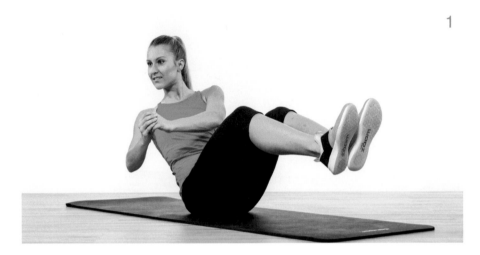

1

Photo 1: Begin in a seated position and raise your legs a few inches off of the floor with your knees bent. Lean back slightly with your upper body and bring your hands together in front of your chest.

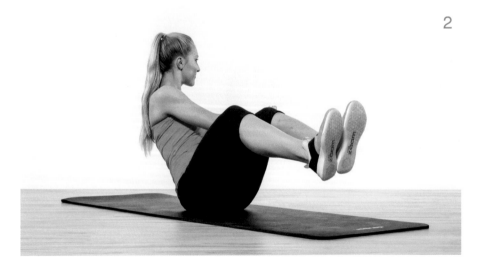

2

Photo 2: Now rotate your upper body from left to right. Your head should turn along with the upper body. Be sure to maintain maximum muscle tension during this exercise.

Prone leg raises ✳

Lower back, gluteals, hip muscles

1

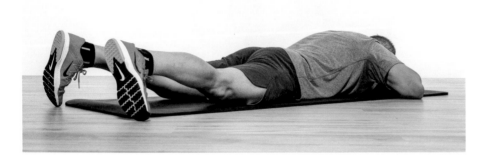

Photo 1: Lie on your stomach on the floor with your arms crossed below your head. Legs should be fully extended.

2

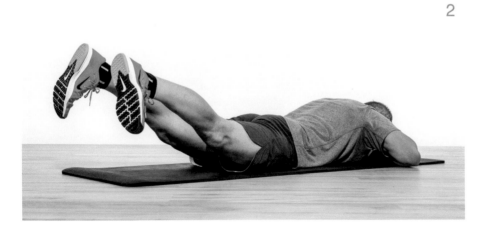

Photo 2: Now lift your extended legs off the floor as high as you can, making sure that your feet are flexed.

Important: the upper body should remain on the floor. The motion is executed strictly from the lower back down. You should hold the position for 1-2 seconds, and lower the legs back down to the starting position. Repeat this motion sequence.

The bug ✳ ✳

Abdominals, lower back, entire trunk

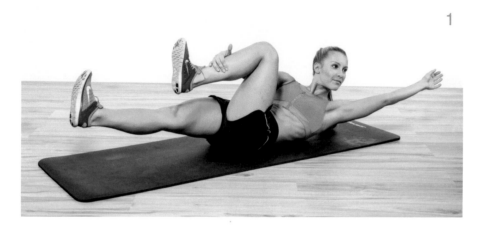

1

Photo 1: Lie on your back on the floor, engaging your abdominal muscles, and slightly raising your shoulders off the floor. Bend the left knee and move it towards the upper body. At the same time, extend the right leg a couple of inches above the floor. Bring your right hand to the left calf and extend the left arm behind you.

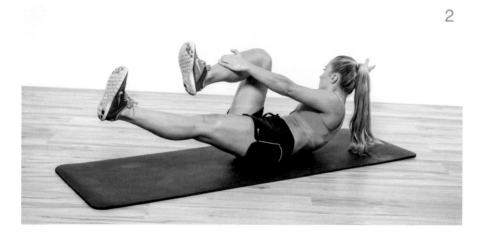

2

Photo 2: Switch sides. Now the left leg should be extended with the right leg simultaneously moving towards the upper body. Then switch arm positions. Keep repeating this motion sequence ensuring that your arms, legs, and shoulders touch the floor.

Alternating prone hip extension with bent knees ✳

Back, gluteals, hip muscles

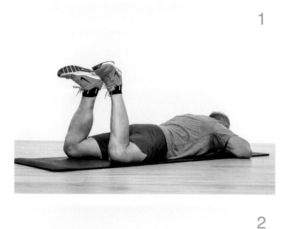

1

Photo 1: Lie on your stomach, on the floor with your arms resting below the head. Legs should mostly be closed with your knees bent so that the calves are in a vertical position.

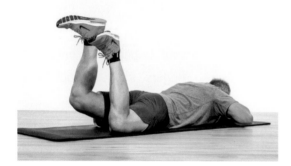

2

Photo 2, Photo 3: Now alternate raising your legs as high as you can. The upper body should rest on the floor and not move. The motion should be executed from the lower back down, without momentum.

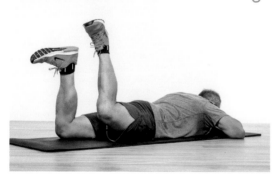

3

Fingers to toes ✳✳✳

Abdominals, lower back, hip muscles

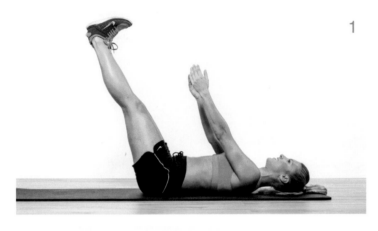

1

Photo 1: This is an exercise for the toughest! Lie on your back on the floor. At first, the upper body should remain on the floor. Now fully extend your legs up at an almost 90-degree angle, as demonstrated in the photo. Fully extend your arms parallel to your legs.

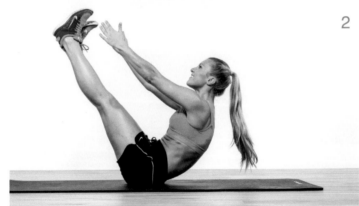

2

Photo 2: Now use your abdominal strength to raise your upper body until your fingers almost touch your toes.

Important: leg position should not change.

A tip from Mike

This is a wonderful exercise to really torture yourself with and get the abs in beach condition. You want to test your limits? Then I would recommend the classic Tabata method: repeat 8 sets of 20 seconds each. Take a 10-second break between sets. Guaranteed sore abs!

Bilateral hip and trunk extension ✳

Entire back, shoulders

1

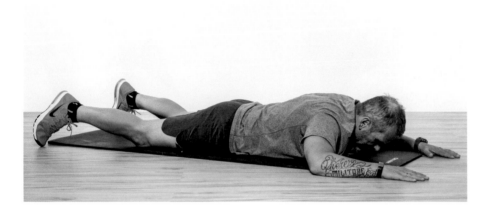

Photo 1: Lie on your stomach on the floor. Extend your legs and arms. Rest them on the floor in order to start, as shown in the photo.

2

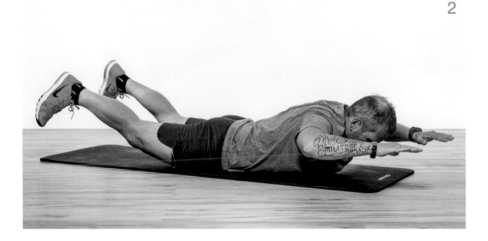

Photo 2: By engaging your core muscles, raise both legs and arms about 2 inches off of the floor. Hold this position for 1-2 seconds and then lower back down. Remember not to allow your arms and legs to touch the floor.

Hands to heels ✳✳

Obliques, core

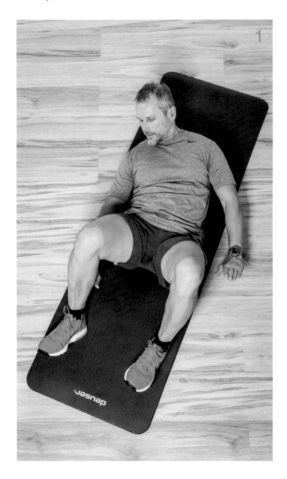 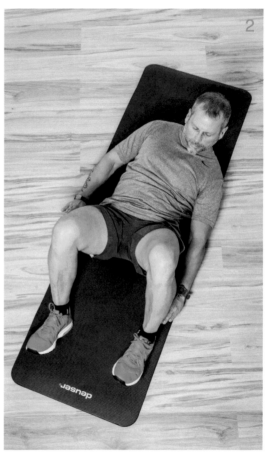

Photo 1, Photo 2: Lie on your back on the floor and bend both knees. Slightly raise your upper body. Arms should be extended forward on the floor close to the body.

Now try to touch your right heel with your right hand and your left heel with your left hand, alternating sides. This exercise primarily works the oblique abdominal muscles.

Plank jacks * *

Core, gluteals, shoulders, abductors, adductors

A near classic whole-body exercise. Get into a forearm plank with your elbows below shoulders. Engage your abdominal muscles.

1

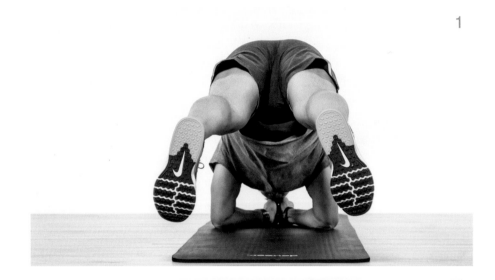

2

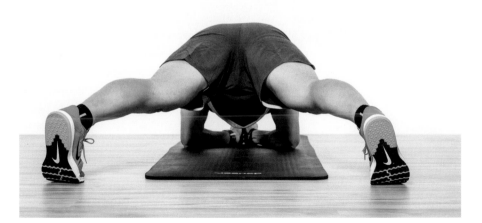

Photo 1, Photo 2: From this position, hop your legs apart as wide as you can and immediately return to the starting position.

Plank knee-up ✳✳✳

Abdominals, lower back, shoulders, chest, iliopsoas muscles

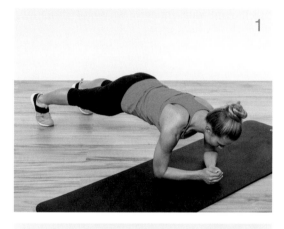

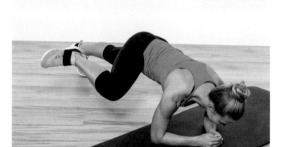

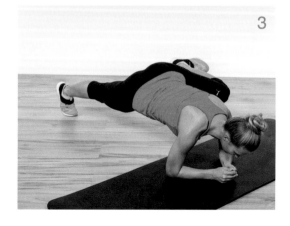

Photo 1: This is also an exercise for almost all muscle groups, however the emphasis is on the core. Begin in a forearm plank with elbows below shoulders.

Photo 2: Now bend the right knee and move it as far as you can towards the elbow. The position of your arm should remain unchanged.

Photo 3: Return to the starting position, the classic forearm plank, and repeat the exercise with the left leg.

Classic sit-up ✳✳

Abdominals, lower back

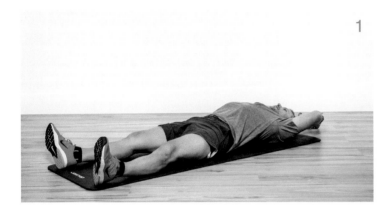

Photo 1: Lie on your back on the floor with legs fully extended. Now raise your arms overhead, on the floor.

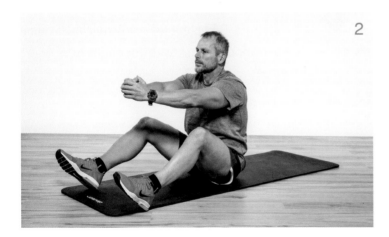

Photo 2: Use your abdominal strength to pull yourself up until you are in a seated position with a straight back. The arms should remain extended during the entire exercise, and in the final position at about chest level.

Variation: if you alternate rotating your trunk about 90 degrees to the right and left as you pull yourself up, you will work the oblique muscles much more.

Boxer crunches ✳✳

Abdominals, lower back, chest, shoulders

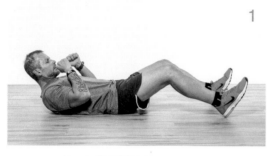

Photo 1: Lie on your back on the floor and raise your upper body a couple of inches. Slightly bend your knees and allow your heels to rest on the floor. Close your hands into fists and hold them at about chest level, as shown in the photo.

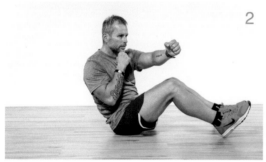

Photo 2: Now use your core muscles to pull yourself up to a seated position. During that motion, your left fist should shoot forward like a boxing punch.

Photo 3: Return to the starting position.

Photo 4: Complete the next crunch. This time you should punch with your right fist.

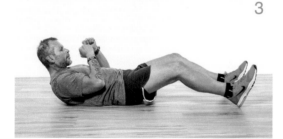

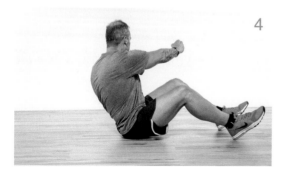

Reverse crunch ✳ ✳ ✳

Abdominals, lower back, shoulders

Photo 1: Lie on your back on the floor and move your legs into a vertical position. Arms should rest on the floor alongside the body.

Photo 2: Use your abdominal strength to raise your pelvis as high as you can off of the floor. Then return to the starting position.

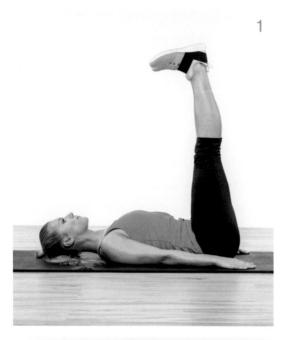

1

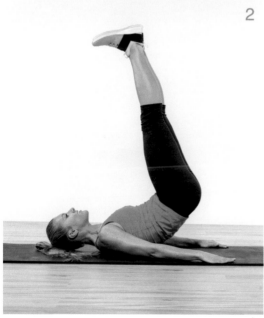

2

Helicopter reverse curl ✳✳✳

The entire core, shoulders

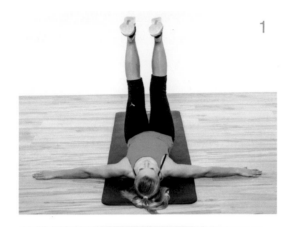

1

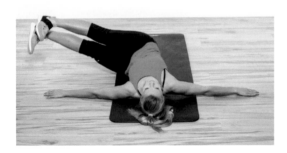

2

Photo 1: Lie on your back on the floor and place your legs in a vertical position so that they form a right angle to your upper body and the floor. Arms should be out to the side at shoulder level, palms down.

Photo 2: Now lower your extended legs as far to the left as possible and hold this position for 1-2 seconds. As you do so, do not change the position of your arms and upper body.

Photo 3: Now slowly move your legs back to the starting position and then lower them to the right side. Briefly hold and then return to the start.

3

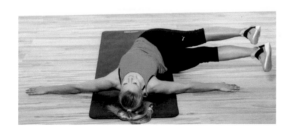

Bicycles ✳ ✳

All abdominal muscles

1

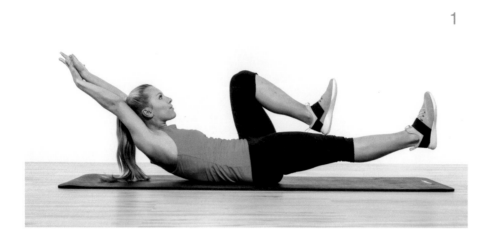

Photo 1: Lie on your back on the floor. Extend your arms overhead and bring your hands together. Slightly raise the upper body. Lift and extend the right leg and move the left knee towards the chest.

2

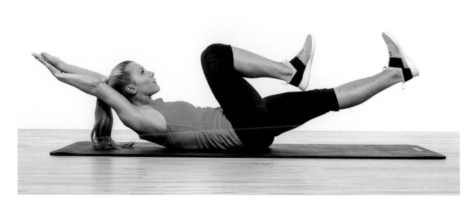

Photo 2: In one fluid motion, extend the left leg and bring the right knee in, and then reverse again like if riding a bike. The position of the upper body should remain lifted during the entire exercise and is not to change.

Bridge ✳ ✳

Lower back, abdominals

1

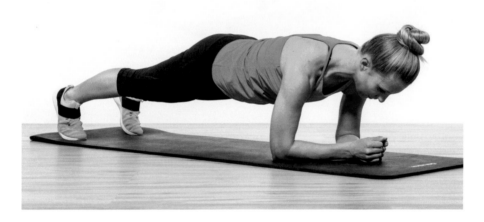

Photo 1: Get into the forearm plank position with elbows below shoulders. Toes should be slightly more than hip-width apart, and upper body and abdominal muscles engaged. The body should form a nearly straight line from heels to the top of the head. Hold this position for 10-120 seconds, depending on your fitness level.

Moving side plank ✳✳

Abdominals, lower back

1

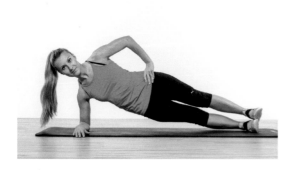

Photo 1: On your side, support yourself on your right forearm with the right elbow below the shoulder. The forearm should point forward and your legs stacked in an extended position, as shown in the photo. The left hand will rest on the left hip. Be sure to engage the gluteal and core muscles.

Photo 2: From this position, lower your pelvis a couple of inches towards the floor.

2

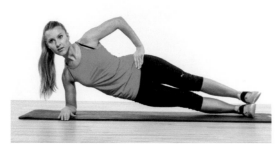

Photo 3: Then lift the pelvis as high as possible, past the starting position. This motion sequence should remain fluid and continuous.

Switch sides after completing one whole set, and support yourself on the left forearm.

3

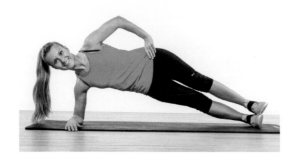

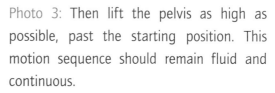

Steady side plank ✳✳✳

Abdominals, lower back, shoulders, iliopsoas muscles

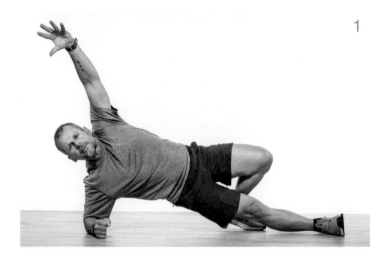

Photo 1: From a side-plank position, extend the left arm overhead and stabilize the body by planting the left foot behind the extended right leg as shown in the photo.

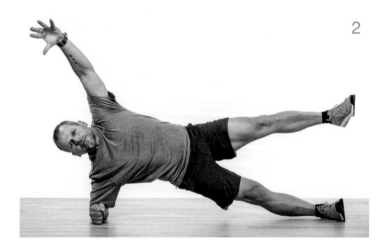

Photo 2: Now lift the left leg parallel to the floor, as shown in the photo. Hold this position 10-30 seconds while maintaining whole-body muscle tension, and switch sides.

Legs

Men often neglect their legs during workouts; however, insufficient legwork can result in muscle imbalances. That is why you should always include leg exercises in your workouts. You will learn an assortment of exercises on the following pages.

Seated leg raises ✳

Quadriceps, hip muscles

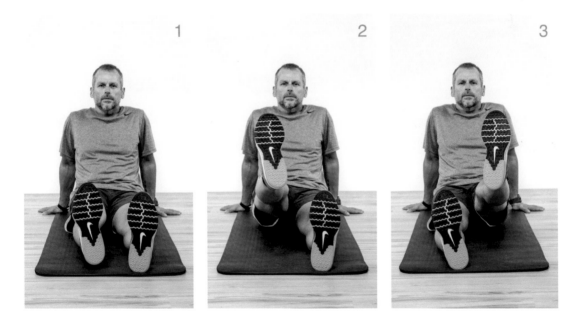

Photo 1: Sit on the floor with your legs extended in front of you, and hands propped on the floor at your sides.

Photo 2, Photo 3: Now lift and lower your right leg.

Important: do not let the leg touch the floor and be sure to maintain muscle tension in your core. The upper body is not to move during this motion sequence. Switch legs after 20-60 seconds.

Single-leg pelvic thrust ✳✳

Hamstring, gluteals

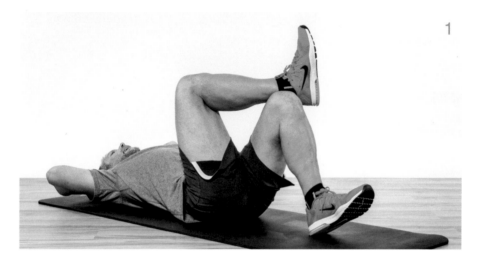

Photo 1: Lie on your back on the floor. Bend the left knee and rest the left heel on the floor. Rest your right calf on your left knee, as shown in the photo.

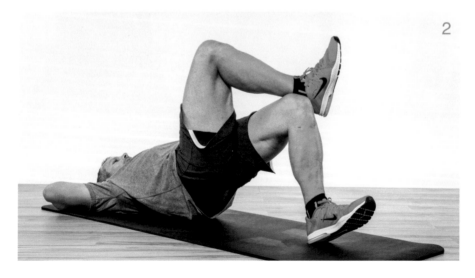

Photo 2: Now push yourself up with your left leg so your thigh, pelvis and upper body form a nearly straight line. Briefly hold this position, and lower down. Complete one whole set with the left leg, and switch to the right leg.

Single-leg lunge ✳✳

All leg muscles

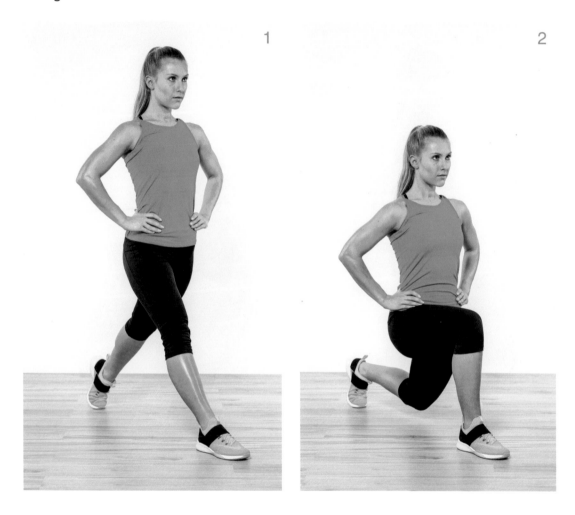

Photo 1: Stand in an astride stance as shown in the photo. Rest your hands on your hips and keep the upper body in an upright position and maintain muscle tension.

Photo 2: Now drop the left knee until your right thigh is parallel to the floor and the left knee almost touches the floor. The position of the upper body should not change. Then return to the starting position.

Here, too, the rule is: complete one set on the right, and then on the left side.

Air squats ✳✳

All thigh muscles

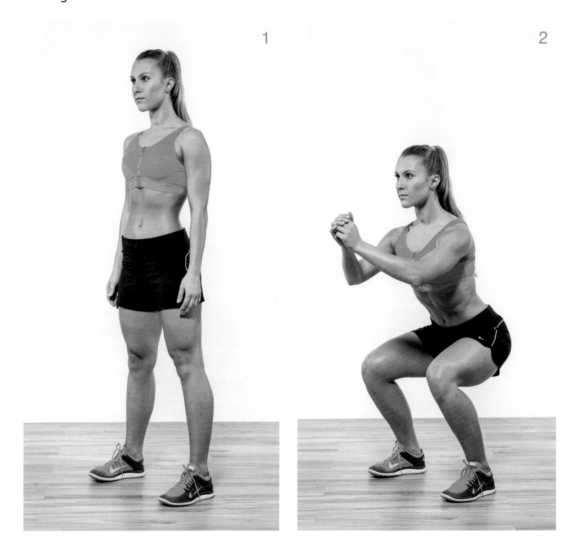

1   2

Photo 1: Stand upright with your feet shoulder-width apart. Arms should hang loosely at your sides.

Photo 2: Now lower your bottom until your thighs are almost 90 degrees to your lower legs. At the same time, bring your arms forward to about chest level. Keep repeating this motion sequence.

Supine single leg raise ✳

Hamstring, iliopsoas muscles

1

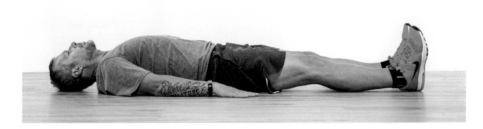

Photo 1: Lie on your back on the floor with both legs extended and arms resting at your sides.

2

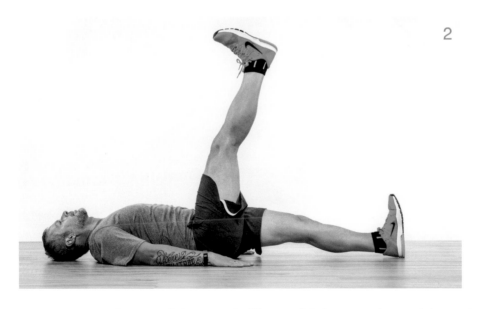

Photo 2: Now raise your right extended leg until it is at an almost right angle to the floor. Then lower the leg back down. Complete one whole set with the right leg, and then switch to the left.

Squat-kick ✳✳

All thigh muscles

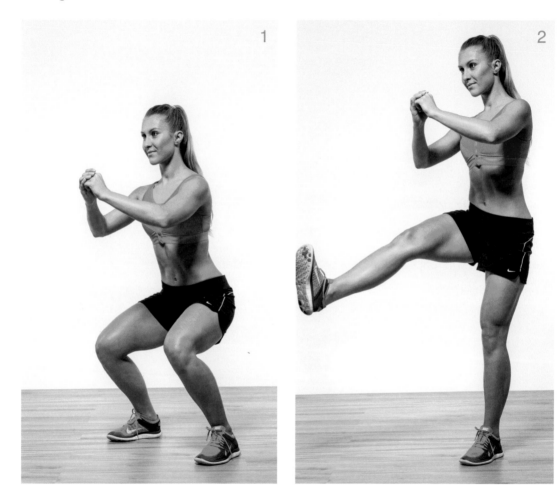

Photo 1: Move into a squat from an upright position. Legs should be about shoulder-width apart, elbows bent, and arms held at chest level.

Photo 2: Now straighten up and raise your extended right leg as high as you can. Then return to a squat position, come up again and perform the kicking motion with your left leg.

Jump lunge ✳✳✳

All leg muscles, gluteals

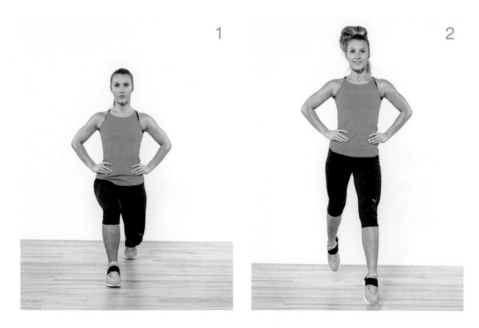

Photo 1: Begin in a classic lunge position, hands on hips and a straight back.

Photo 2: Now jump up with both legs.

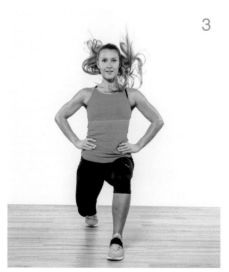

Photo 3: Land in a lunge, this time with the other leg. During the jumps, the upper body should remain as still as possible. Focus on core stability during landings.

Jump squats ✳✳

All leg muscles, gluteals

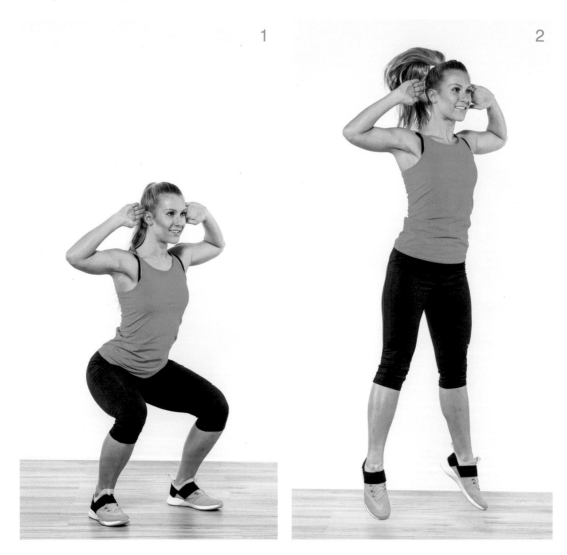

Photo 1: Move into a classic squat position. Place your hands behind your head.

Important: maintain high body tension.

Photo 2: Now forcefully push off the floor with both legs and land back in a squat. Arms remain folded behind the head.

Rotational squats ✻✻

All leg muscles, abdominals, lower back

1

2

3

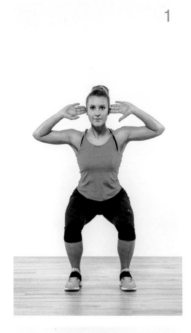
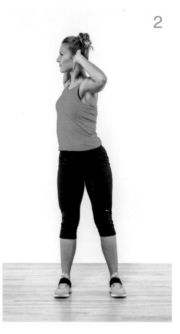
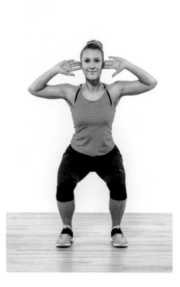

4

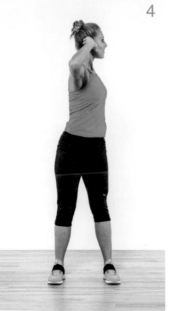

Photo 1: Begin in the same squat position as the previous exercise. Fingers should rest against the side of the head.

Photo 2: Now come to an upright position while rotating your upper body to the right.

Photo 3: Return to a squat position.

Photo 4: Rotate in the opposite direction.

Jack squat ✳

All thigh muscles, gluteals

1   2

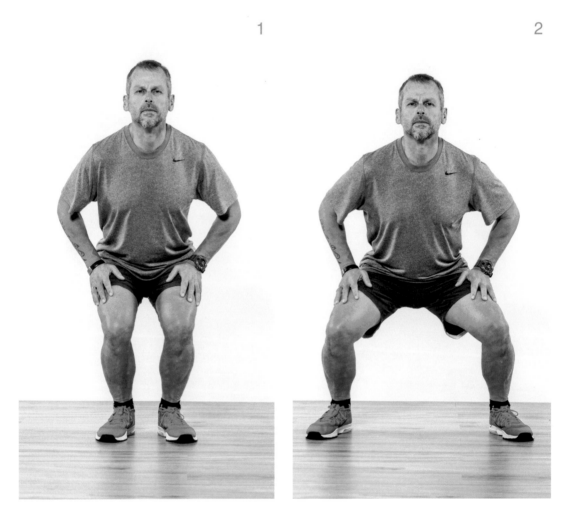

Photo 1: Stand with your feet shoulder-width apart. Bend your knees as shown in the photo. Hands should rest on your thighs. Engage your abdominal muscles and bend slightly forward with the upper body.

Photo 2: Jump into a slightly wider stance with both legs. Then jump back into the starting position. Because the abdominal muscles are engaged, the upper body should remain steady and motionless during the jumps.

Side-lying hip abduction ✳✳

Iliopsoas muscles, gluteals

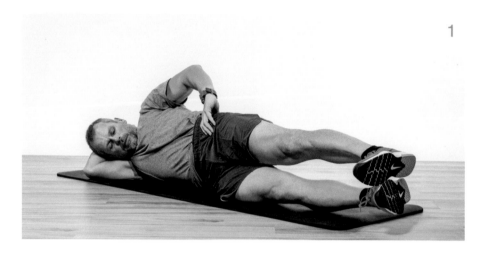

Photo 1: Lie on your right side and rest your head on your arm. Legs should be stacked.

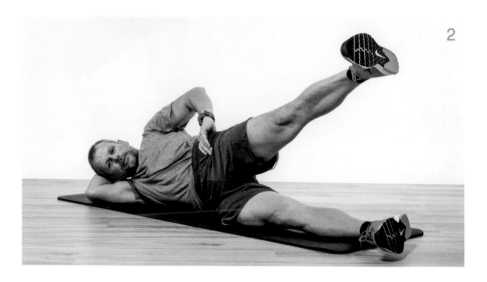

Photo 2: Slowly and steadily raise and lower the left leg without allowing it to touch the floor. Be sure to maintain body tension.

Here, too, the rule is: switch sides after completing one whole set.

Jack squat with arm action ✳✳

All thigh muscles, shoulders

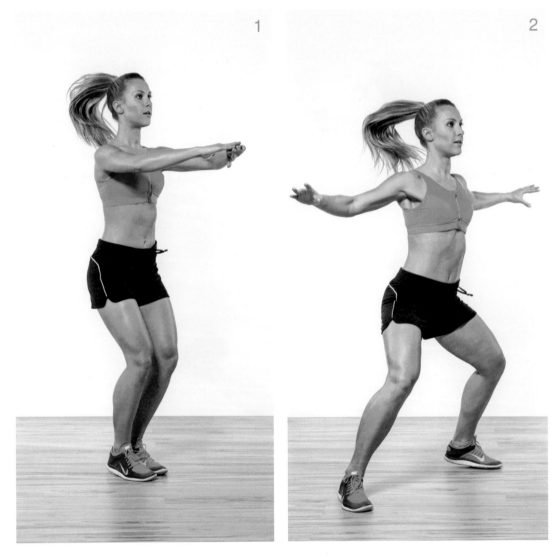

Photo 1: Starting position should be a closed stance, with knees slightly bent, and arms extended forward at chest level.

Photo 2: Vigorously jump with both legs into a straddle. Simultaneously swing the extended arms to the sides and immediately jump back into the starting position.

Bridge with lateral leg-raise ✳✳

All thigh muscles, shoulders, gluteals

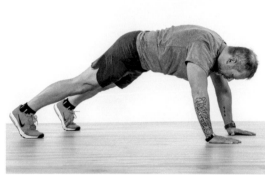

Photo 1: Get down on all fours so your body forms a bridge. Arms and legs should be extended.

Photo 2: From this position, raise your left leg to the side as high as you can, as shown in the photo.

Photo 3: Return to the starting position and execute the same motion with the right leg.

Important: maintain significant whole-body tension.

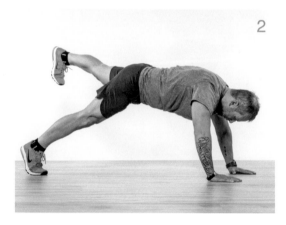

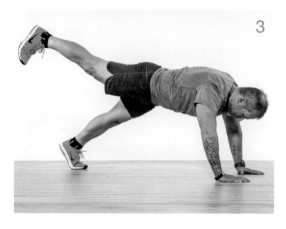

Static squat with scissor arms ✳

All thigh muscles, shoulders

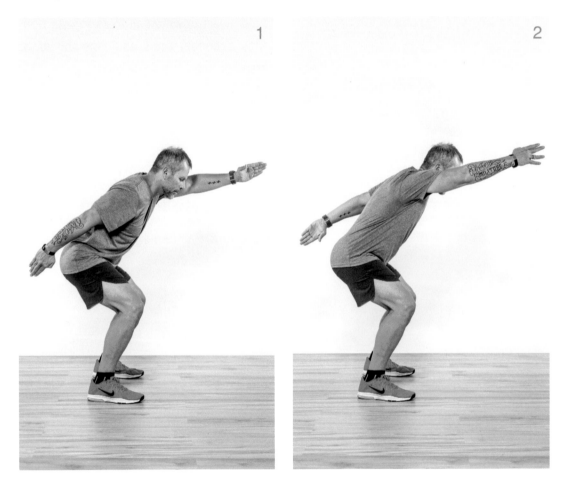

Photo 1, Photo 2: Bend your knees as much as possible to move into a squat position. Lean slightly forward with the upper body and keep your back straight. Now move your arms forward and back, alternating arms. Make sure your thigh and core muscles are engaged throughout the exercise.

Back lunge with forward kick ✳✳

All thigh muscles, gluteals, iliopsoas muscles

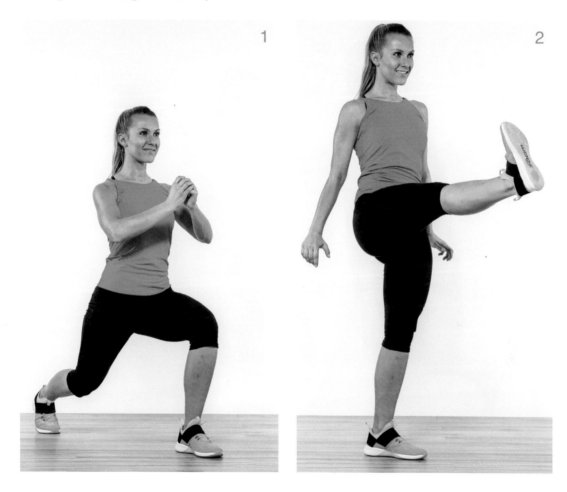

Photo 1: Take a big step back with your right leg while keeping the upper body steady and straight. The left thigh and lower leg should be at a right angle to each other. Bring your hands together in front of the chest.

Photo 2: Now swing the extended right leg forward and up as high as you can. Then repeat the motion sequence with the left leg.

Calf raises ✳

Calves

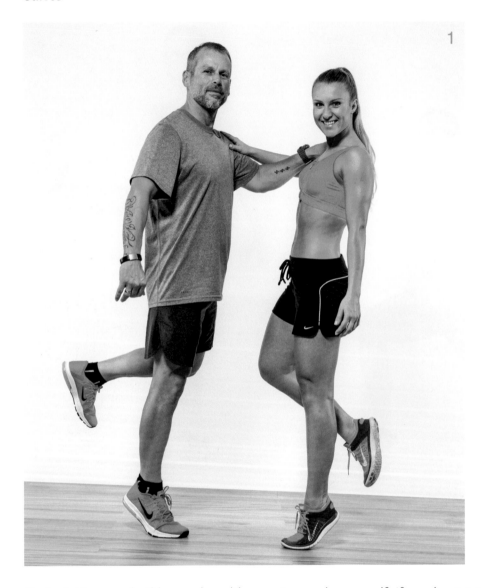

Photo 1: You can do this exercise with a partner or by yourself. If you have trouble keeping your balance, try supporting yourself against a wall. Begin in an upright position and push up onto your toes so that your heels lift off of the floor as high as possible. Briefly hold this position and lower your heels back down.

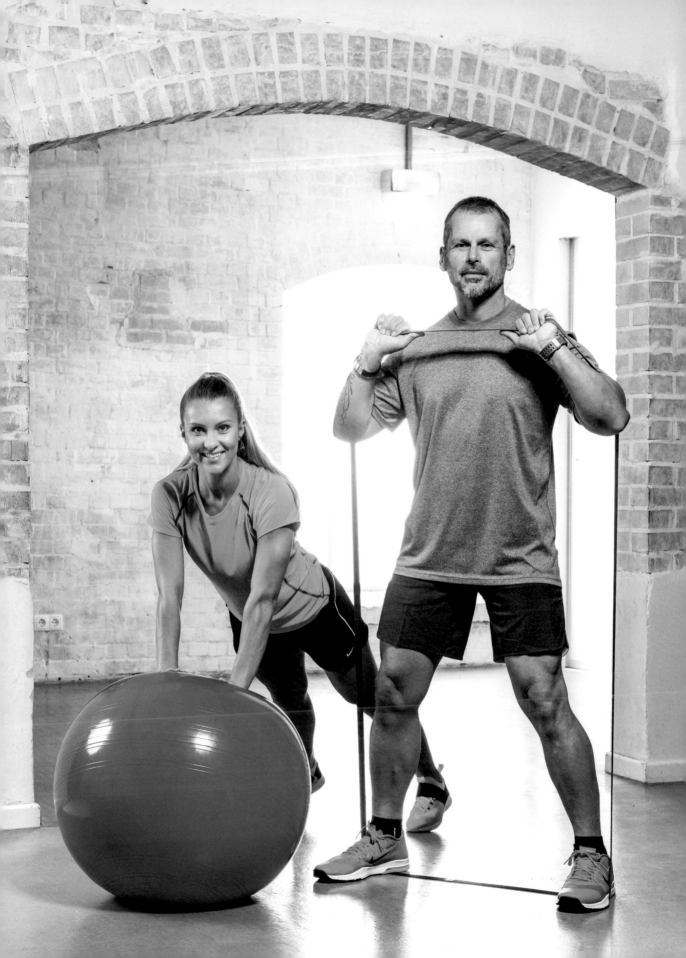

9 CIRCUIT TRAINING – GET FIT WITH POINTS!

On the following pages, you will learn 15 different circuits that you can use to make your workouts flexible and versatile. All of the exercises will be taken from previous chapters so may seem familiar.

The brilliant thing is that you will receive points for each workout based on the number of sets you complete. At the end of the week, the point system on page 187 will help you review how well and effectively you have trained. There are minimum scores that should be achieved based on your fitness level and athletic goals. A nice side benefit is that it is a great way to compete against friends. Who will be the one with the most points this week?

As always, one thing is important. Everyone trains and scores at their own level which means that if you classify yourself as a beginner and complete the respective duration and number of repetitions per exercise, you will receive the same number of points as the pro that has to perform each exercise for a longer period of time. You decide which workout level is right for you and which demands are appropriate for your physical condition.

All of the circuits in this book are marked with the number of points for the respective number of sets. Record the number of points you scored after each training unit (ideally in our fitness training journal), and add them up at the end of the week. You can then look at the chart and use these to see how much you did for your body.

Important: the circuits on the following pages are merely suggestions. Once you are familiar with the individual exercises you can design countless circuits of your own.

CIRCUIT TRAINING – GET FIT WITH POINTS!
Weekly check-in – will I become Mr. or Mrs. Six-pack?

Record your points earned after every workout and add them up at the end of each training week. After seven days, this will give you your total points. You can use the following chart to classify your performance.

< 80 points:	Flu? Get well soon!
85-120 points:	The chapter on motivation begins on page 52. Please read!
125-210 points:	You are on your way – but not at your goal!
215-300 points:	Solid – with room to grow!
305-400 points:	Above average – is it enough?
405-600 points:	Respect – your body thanks you!
605-800 points:	Who is that bastard?
805-1000 points:	Mr./Ms. Six-pack
> 1000 points:	Freak! Is exercise all you think about?

Basic workout (Bodyweight)

A circuit of eight bodyweight exercises. You will cover all muscle groups and complete one set in just a few minutes. Instructions for repetitions always refer to one side of the body.

1) Hands to heels

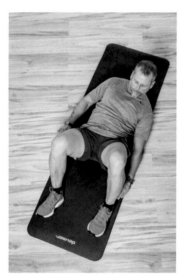

Begin with a classic abdominal exercise that also significantly works the oblique abdominal muscles. Description on page 156.

Continue with:
Exercise 2, Bridge. ➡

Beginners 5 repetitions, Intermediates 10 repetitions, **Pros 15 repetitions**

2) Bridge

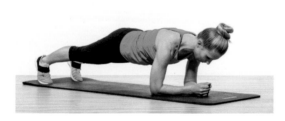

A classic, also called "plank." Strengthens the entire core. Page 164.

Continue with:
Exercise 3, Back lunge with forward kick. ➡

Beginners 10 seconds, Intermediates 15 seconds, **Pros 20 seconds**

3) Back lunge with forward kick

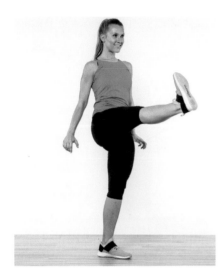

After working the abs, it's time for a leg workout. Good for all thigh muscles and flexibility. Page 181.

Continue with:
Exercise 4, Jump squats. ➡

Beginners 5 repetitions, Intermediates 10 repetitions, **Pros 15 repetitions**

4) Jump squats

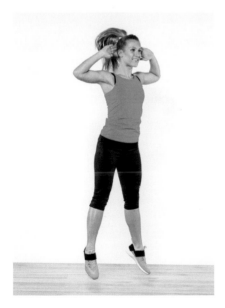

After a while, you'll really feel your legs. Also challenging with respect to endurance. Page 174.

Weiter geht es mit:
Exercise 5, Triangle pushups. ➡

Beginners 5 repetitions, Intermediates 10 repetitions, **Pros 15 repetitions**

5) Triangle pushups

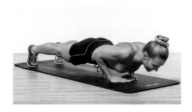

Brutal effort – but triceps, chest, and shoulders love it. Perfect for the upper body. Page 137.

Continue with:
Exercise 6, Floor row. ➡

Beginners 5 repetitions, Intermediates 10 repetitions, **Pros 15 repetitions**

6) Floor row

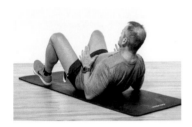

Hugely effective for working the latissimus dorsi, Page 142.

Continue with:
Exercise 7, High knees. ➡

Beginners 5 repetitions, Intermediates 10 repetitions, **Pros 15 repetitions**

7) High knees

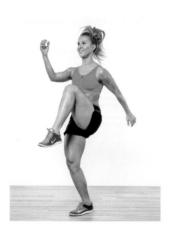

Homestretch! Great for the legs, gluteals, and core – and endurance. Page 128.

Continue with:
Exercise 8, Mountain climbers. ➡

Beginners 5 repetitions, Intermediates 10 repetitions, **Pros 15 repetitions**

8) Mountain climbers

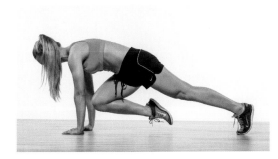

The final exercise – it packs a wallop because it works the entire body. Page 131.

Beginners 5 repetitions, Intermediates 10 repetitions, **Pros 15 repetitions**

Congratulations! You have completed the basic circuit!

A tip from Mike

Can you complete the pro version of the basic circuit without a problem? Then check out the Tabata method. You should do every exercise for 20 seconds with a 10-second break in-between. Take a 1-minute break between sets. I promise you will be panting no later than the third set!

Get fit with points! ✳ ✳ ✳

One set = 10 points
Two sets, 90 seconds break between sets = 25 points
Three sets, 90 seconds break between sets = 45 points
Four sets, 90 seconds break between sets = 70 points
Five sets = 90 seconds break between sets = 100 points
Six sets = 90 seconds break between sets = 150 points
Seven sets = 90 seconds break between sets = 200 points

No Excuses workout (Bodyweight)

As the name suggests, no excuses allowed! The increasing repetitions make this circuit considerably more difficult than the previous one. It combines exercises for all parts of the body and perfectly unites strength and endurance components.

1) Burpees

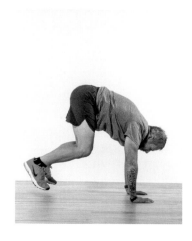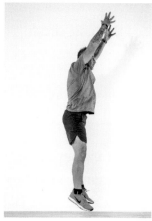

This killer exercise up front. Burpees push everyone to their limit. They work the entire body. Description on page 126.

Continue with:
Exercise 2, Classic pushups. ➡

Beginners 5 repetitions, Intermediates 10 repetitions, **Pros 15 repetitions**

2) Classic pushups

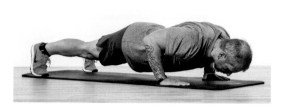

The next whole-body exercise. Make sure your execution is clean and controlled, and your back straight. Page 136.

Continue with:
Exercise 3, Jump lunges. ➡

Beginners 10 repetitions, Intermediates 15 repetitions, **Pros 20 repetitions**

3) Jump lunges

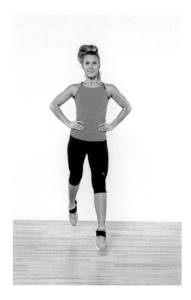

Perfect for legs and gluteals while also requiring lots of coordination, and challenging with respect to endurance. Page 173.

Continue with:
Exercise 4, Air squats. ➡

Beginners 15 repetitions, **Intermediates 20 repetitions**, **Pros 30 repetitions**

4) Air squats

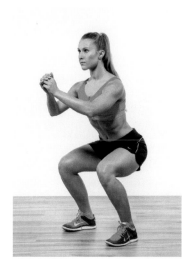

Again legs and gluteals. Really works the thighs. Page 170.

Continue with:
Exercise 5, Dynamic sit-ups. ➡

Beginners 20 repetitions, **Intermediates 30 repetitions**, **Pros 40 repetitions**

5) Dynamic sit-ups

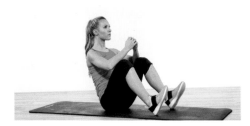

Time to work the abdominals. The number of repetitions is pretty steep. Tough it out! Page 148.

Continue with:
Exercise 6, Mountain climbers. ➡

Beginners 20 repetitions, **Intermediates 40 repetitions**, **Pros 60 repetitions**

6) Mountain climbers

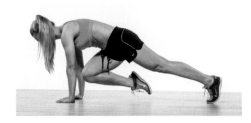

Another whole-body exercise that challenges your stamina. Remember that the number of repetitions is per leg! Page 131.

Continue with:
Exercise 7, High knees. ➡

Beginners 30 repetitions, **Intermediates 50 repetitions**, **Pros 80 repetitions**

7) High knees

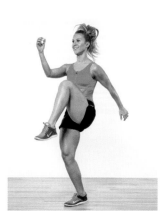

At this point you will have to fight. Your body will be grateful for the effort, seriously! Page 128.

Continue with:
Exercise 8, Jumping jacks. ➡

Beginners 40 repetitions, **Intermediates 60 repetitions**, **Pros 90 repetitions**

8) Jumping jacks

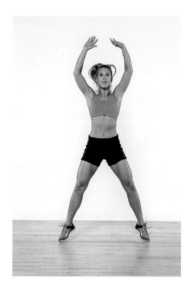

The final exercise, the infamous jumping jacks. Fantastic for legs, gluteals, core, and shoulders.

Beginners 50 repetitions, **Intermediates 100 repetitions**, **Pros 120 repetitions**

Did you tough it out? Well done, because the No Excuses circuit is really tough. What makes it particularly tough is the Get-fit-with-points system (see below). Because you only earn lots of points if you complete several sets.

Get fit with points! ✳✳✱

One set = 15 points

Two sets, 90 seconds break between sets = 35 points

Three sets, 90 seconds break between sets = 60 points

Four sets, 90 seconds break between sets = 90 points

Five sets = 90 seconds break between sets = 135 points

Six sets = 90 seconds break between sets = 170 points

Seven sets = 90 seconds break between sets = 200 points

Tabata workout (Bodyweight)

You are already familiar with the Tabata workout method. Load phases and breaks alternate at a 2:1 ratio. That means that you work out 20 seconds, take a 10-second break, then do the next exercise for 20 seconds, etc. You work out for a total of 8 x 20 seconds. That means one Tabata set takes four minutes to complete.

In this circuit, you complete four Tabatas back to back. Then you will have completed one set. If you want to earn 250 points at the end, you must complete all of the Tabatas five times in a row. You will take 60-second breaks between individual Tabatas, and 90 second between sets.

Tabata A

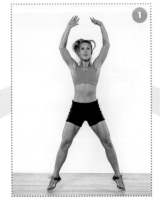

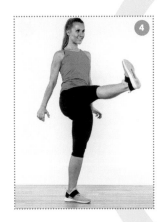

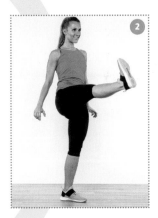

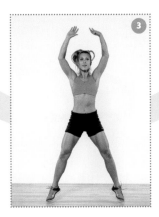

1. Jumping jacks (2 x 20 seconds), page 129

2. Back lunge with forward kick (2 x 20 seconds), page 181

3. Jumping jacks (2 x 20 seconds)

4. Back lunge with forward kick (2 x 20 seconds)

Tabata B

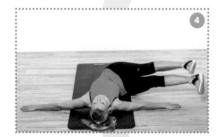

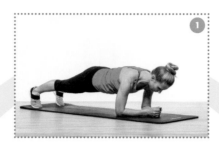

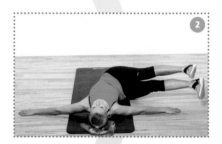

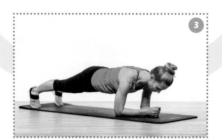

① Bridge (2 x 20 seconds), page 164

② Helicopter reverse curls (2 x 20 seconds), page 162

③ Bridge (2 x 20 seconds)

④ Helicopter reverse curls (2 x 20 seconds)

Tabata C

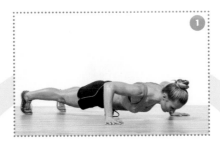

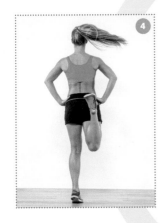

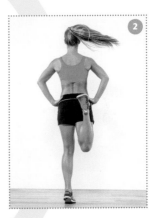

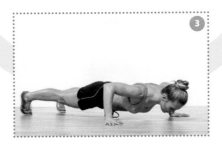

1 Wide-grip pushups (2 x 20 seconds), page 138

2 Butt kicks (2 x 20 seconds), page 130

3 Wide-grip pushups (2 x 20 seconds)

4 Butt kicks (2 x 20 seconds)

Tabata D

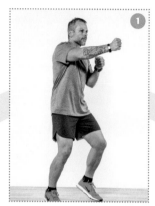

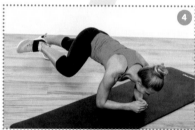

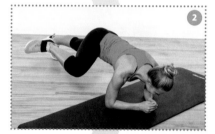

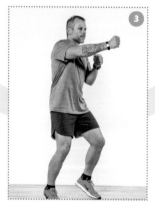

1 Shadowboxing (2 x 20 seconds), page 132

2 Plank knee-up (2 x 20 seconds), page 158

3 Shadowboxing (2 x 20 seconds)

4 Plank knee-up (2 x 20 seconds)

Get fit with points! ✳✳✳

One set = 30 points

Two sets, 90 seconds break between sets = 70 points

Three sets, 90 seconds break between sets = 120 points

Four sets, 90 seconds break between sets = 180 points

Five sets = 90 seconds break between sets = 250 points

Mixed workout I
(Bodyweight, exercise band)

The first mixed circuit – this time you will use the exercise band (Deuser band) in addition to your bodyweight. The focus is again on a combination of endurance and strength training.

1) High knees

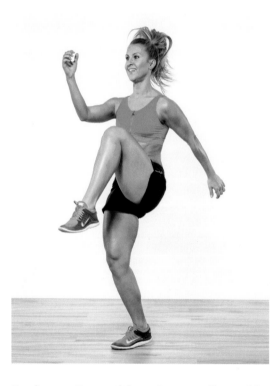

A whole-body and endurance exercise to start. Description on page 128.

Continue with:
Exercise 2, Bicep curls. ➡

Beginners 5 repetitions, **Intermediates 10 repetitions**, **Pros 15 repetitions**

2) Bicep curls (with the band)

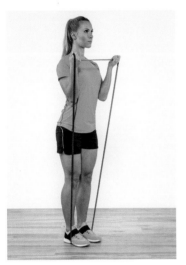

Want strong arms? Then work your biceps! The exercise band is perfect for this exercise. Page 91.

Continue with:
Exercise 3, High knees. ➡

Beginners 10 repetitions, Intermediates 15 repetitions, **Pros 20 repetitions**

3) High knees

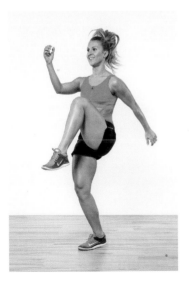

Get those knees up as fast and vigorously as possible! Page 128.

Continue with:
Exercise 4, Standing chest press. ➡

Beginners 5 repetitions, Intermediates 10 repetitions, **Pros 15 repetitions**

4) Standing chest press

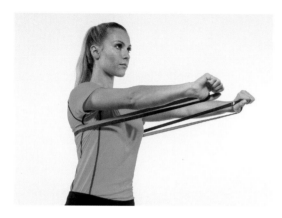

This exercise shapes the entire upper body, particularly the chest. Page 88.

Continue with:
Exercise 5, Butt kicks. ➡

Beginners 10 repetitions, Intermediates 15 repetitions, **Pros 20 repetitions**

5) Butt kicks

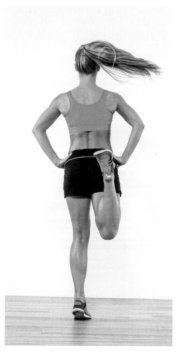

Rapidly pull your heels towards your bottom, alternating legs. The number of repetitions again is per side. Page 130.

Continue with:
Übung 6, Frontdrücken. ➡

Beginners 5 repetitions, Intermediates 10 repetitions, **Pros 15 repetitions**

6) Overhead press

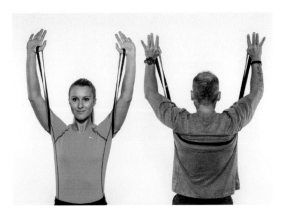

Grab your Deuser band! This time the focus is on shoulders. Page 85.

Continue with:

Exercise 7, Butt kicks. ➡

Beginners 10 repetitions, Intermediates 15 repetitions, **Pros 20 repetitions**

7) Butt Kicks

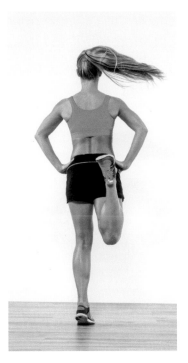

Second set of butt kicks. They work the entire thigh musculature. Page 130.

Continue with:

Exercise 8, Leg press. ➡

Beginners 5 repetitions, Intermediates 10 repetitions, **Pros 15 repetitions**

8) Leg press

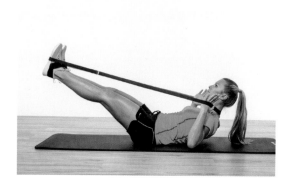

The final exercise, because you have successfully completed the first set of this circuit. One more leg workout. Page 102.

Beginners 10 repetitions, Intermediates 15 repetitions, **Pros 20 repetitions**

Get fit with points! ✳✳✱
One set = 10 points
Two sets, 90 seconds break between sets = 25 points
Three sets, 90 seconds break between sets = 45 points
Four sets, 90 seconds break between sets = 70 points
Five sets = 90 seconds break between sets = 100 points
Six sets = 90 seconds break between sets = 150 points
Seven sets = 90 seconds break between sets = 200 points

Mixed workout II (Bodyweight, stability ball)

Another mixed circuit – this time bodyweight and stability ball exercises. Again the focus is on endurance and strength, with particular emphasis on abdominals and lower back.

1) Jumping jacks

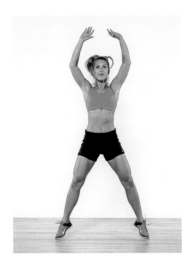

Get your blood moving! Jumping jacks are the perfect choice! Page 129.

Continue with:
Exercise 2, Pushups on the ball. ➡

Beginners 10 repetitions, **Intermediates 20 repetitions**, **Pros 30 repetitions**

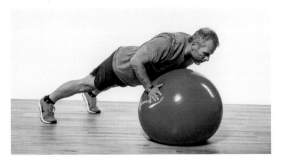

2) Pushups on the ball

A brutal exercise. Due to the ball's instability, the arms, shoulders, chest, and back must work even harder. Page 70.

Continue with:
Exercise 3, The bug. ➡

Beginners 5 repetitions, **Intermediates 10 repetitions**, **Pros 15 repetitions**

3) The bug

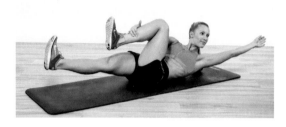

A classic abdominal exercise. Arms and legs move on a diagonal. Page 152.

Continue with:
Exercise 4, Ball-roller. ➡

Beginners 10 repetitions, Intermediates 20 repetitions, **Pros 30 repetitions**

4) Ball-roller

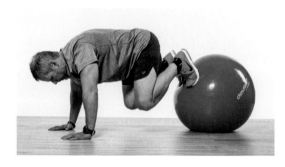

This exercise also works the entire core. Focus on maximum stability. Page 69.

Continue with:
Exercise 5, High knees. ➡

Beginners 5 repetitions, Intermediates 10 repetitions, **Pros 15 repetitions**

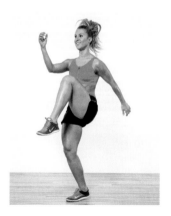

5) High knees

Loosening up the legs, heating up the body. The number of repetitions again refers to one side. Page 128.

Continue with:
Exercise 6, Jackknife with the ball. ➡

Beginners 10 repetitions, Intermediates 20 repetitions, **Pros 30 repetitions**

6) Jackknife with the ball

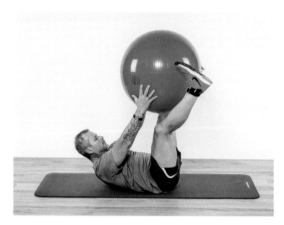

This exercise is similarly difficult with or without the ball. It really gets the abdominals to burn. Page 73.

Continue with:

Exercise 7, Burpees. ➡

Beginners 5 repetitions, Intermediates 10 repetitions, **Pros 15 repetitions**

7) Burpees

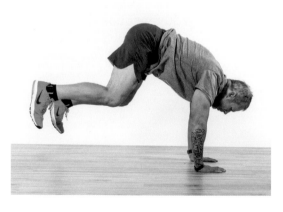

The fat killer – particularly demanding at the end of the circuit. Page 126.

Continue with:

Exercise 8, Russian twist. ➡

Beginners 3 repetitions, Intermediates 5 repetitions, **Pros 8 repetitions**

8) Russian Twist (with ball)

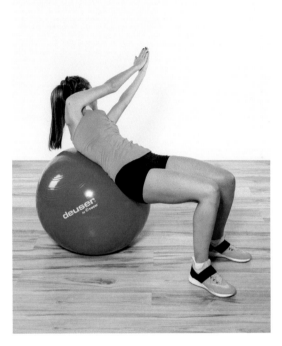

The final exercise – the core is working again, especially the abdominals. Page 71.

Beginners 10 repetitions, Intermediates 20 repetitions, **Pros 30 repetitions**

Get fit with points! ✳✳✳

One set = 15 points

Two sets, 90 seconds break between sets = 35 points

Three sets, 90 seconds break between sets = 60 points

Four sets, 90 seconds break between sets = 90 points

Five sets = 90 seconds break between sets = 135 points

Six sets = 90 seconds break between sets = 170 points

Seven sets = 90 seconds break between sets = 200 points

Strong upper body workout (Bodyweight, free weights)

Eight exercises for a strong upper body – alternating between bodyweight and free weights. Sore muscles guaranteed!

1) Lateral raises

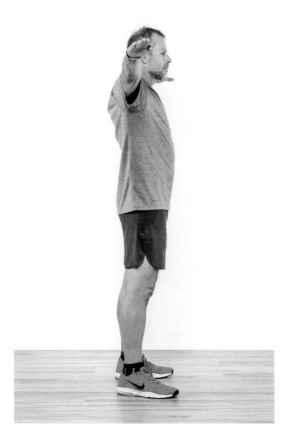

A gentle start to this circuit. However, you will feel 30 repetitions. Emphasis is on the shoulders. Page 145.

Continue with:
Exercise 2, Biceps curls. ➡

Beginners 10 repetitions, **Intermediates 20 repetitions**, **Pros 30 repetitions**

2) Biceps curls

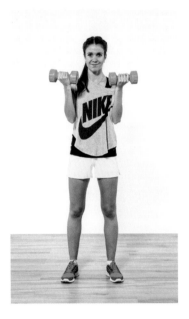

One of the most masculine exercises of all – but also good for women! Shapes the biceps muscles perfectly. Page 107.

Continue with:
Exercise 3, Pushups with core rotation. ➡

Beginners 10 repetitions, **Intermediates 15 repetitions**, **Pros 20 repetitions**

3) Pushups with core rotation

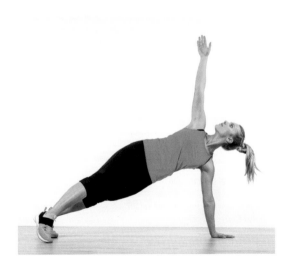

Pushups alone are arduous. Core rotations amplify the effect on the upper body. As always, the number of repetitions refers to just one side. Page 140.

Continue with:
Exercise 4, Reclined triceps press. ➡

Beginners 5 repetitions, **Intermediates 10 repetitions**, **Pros 15 repetitions**

4) Reclined triceps press

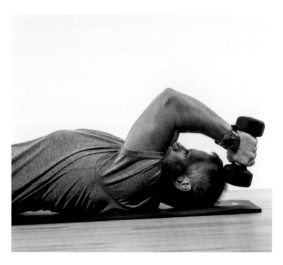

After the biceps, it's time to work the antagonist. The triceps are even more important to a visibly strong upper arm. Page 110.

Continue with:
Exercise 5, Floor row. ➡

Beginners 10 repetitions, Intermediates 15 repetitions, **Pros 20 repetitions**

5) Floor row

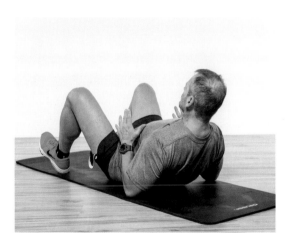

Hugely effective for the upper back. You will really feel those last few repetitions. Page 142.

Continue with:
Exercise 6, Dumbbell shoulder press. ➡

Beginners 10 repetitions, Intermediates 20 repetitions, **Pros 30 repetitions**

6) Dumbbell shoulder press

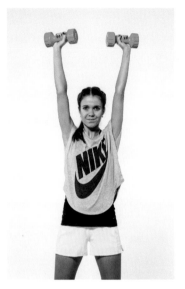

Classic free-weight exercise for strong shoulders. Make sure your movements are slow and controlled. Page 118.

Continue with:
Exercise 7, Triceps kickbacks. ➡

Beginners 10 repetitions, **Intermediates 15 repetitions**, **Pros 20 repetitions**

7) Triceps kickbacks

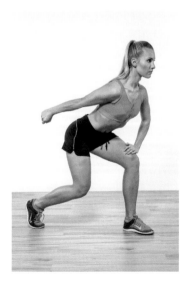

Do you think this looks easy? After no more than 20 reps per side, your triceps will feel as firm as a tennis-ball. Page 135.

Continue with:
Exercise 8, Dumbbell swing. ➡

Beginners 20 repetitions, **Intermediates 30 repetitions**, **Pros 40 repetitions**

8) Dumbbell swing

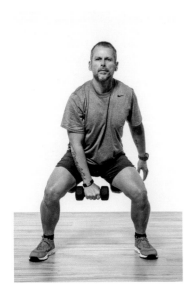

In addition to the shoulders, this also works the legs because of the squats. Again, the number of repetitions refers to just one side. Page 117. You have now completed the first set of this circuit. Awesome!

Beginners 10 repetitions, Intermediates 20 repetitions, **Pros 30 repetitions**

Get fit with points! ✳✳✳

One set = 25 points

Two sets, 90 seconds break between sets = 50 points

Three sets, 90 seconds break between sets = 100 points

Four sets, 90 seconds break between sets = 150 points

Five sets = 90 seconds break between sets = 200 points

Strong legs workout (Bodyweight, free weights)

The combination of the following eight exercises primarily focus on legs and gluteal muscles. You will definitely feel your thighs no later than the third set. Can you handle five sets? Impressive, you collect 200 points!

1) Jack squats

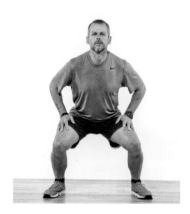

Short and dynamic jumps into a straddle accompanied by a squat. Page 176.

Continue with:
Exercise 2, Squats with weights. ➡

Beginners 15 repetitions, Intermediates 20 repetitions, **Pros 30 repetitions**

2) Squats with weights

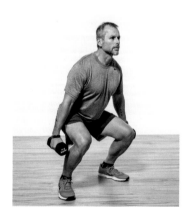

No break for the thighs. Few exercises are as effective for both fat burning and muscle building as squats. The free weights make it twice as tough. Page 115.

Continue with:
Übung 3, Air Squats. ➡

Beginners 10 repetitions, Intermediates 20 repetitions, **Pros 30 repetitions**

3) Air squats

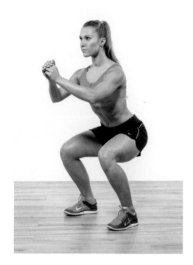

A squat works up to 400 muscles. Regardless of your current workout level, you should definitely feel your legs by now. Page 170.

Continue with:
Exercise 4, Squat with shoulder press. ➡

Beginners 20 repetitions, Intermediates 30 repetitions, **Pros 40 repetitions**

4) Squat with shoulder press

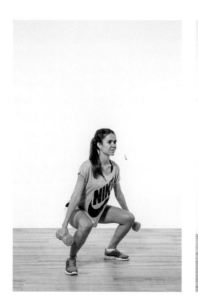
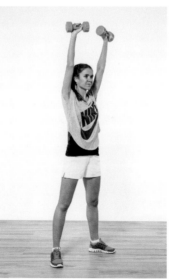

Are your thighs trembling? Suck it up! Adding the shoulder press will allow you to simultaneously work the upper body. Page 116.

Continue with:
Exercise 5, Calf-raises. ➡

Beginners 5 repetitions, Intermediates 10 repetitions, **Pros 15 repetitions**

5) Calf-raises

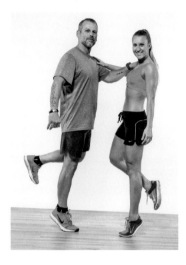

A short break for the thighs where you will work the calves instead. Page 182.

Continue with:
Exercise 6, High knees. ➡

Beginners 20 repetitions, **Intermediates 30 repetitions**, **Pros 40 repetitions**

6) High knees

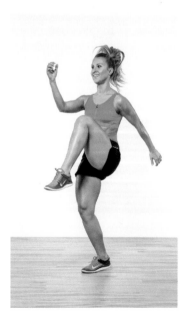

The (per side) repetitions will torture your legs and also challenge your stamina. Try to perform this exercise as vigorously as possible. Page 128.

Continue with:
Exercise 7, Lunges with weights. ➡

Beginners 20 repetitions, **Intermediates 30 repetitions**, **Pros 40 repetitions**

7) Lunges with weights

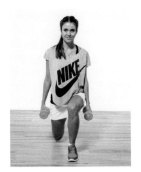

Feel like some extra torture? Then do the repetitions first with the left leg and then switch to the right leg. Page 114.

Continue with:
Exercise 8, Shadowboxing. ➡

Beginners 5 repetitions, Intermediates 10 repetitions, **Pros 15 repetitions**

8) Shadowboxing

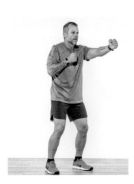

The repetitions refer to the arm movement, meaning the punches (per side). Simultaneously bob and weave to loosen up your leg muscles. Page 132.

Beginners 20 repetitions, Intermediates 30 repetitions, **Pros 40 repetitions**

Get fit with points! ✻✻✻
One set = 40 points
Two sets, 90 seconds break between sets = 80 points
Three sets, 90 seconds break between sets = 120 points
Four sets, 90 seconds break between sets = 160 points
Five sets = 90 seconds break between sets = 200 points

Mixed workout III
(Exercise band, stability ball, free weights)

A classic whole-body circuit. You work legs, upper body, and core. Exercises alternate using exercise bands, ball and free weights.

1) Boxing (with band)

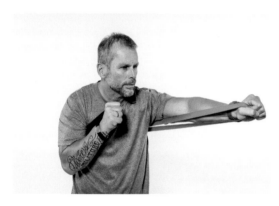

Let's start with shoulders and arms. You can also bob and weave as you do this one. Page 94.

Continue with:
Exercise 2, Rotational lunge with ball. ➡

Beginners 10 repetitions, Intermediates 20 repetitions, **Pros 30 repetitions**

2) Rotational lunge with ball

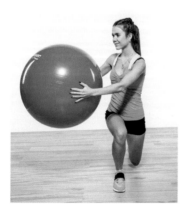

By holding the ball in front of your body, you will work the entire upper body in addition to the legs. Page 72.

Continue with:
Exercise 3, Hammer curls. ➡

Beginners 10 repetitions, Intermediates 15 repetitions, **Pros 20 repetitions**

3) Hammer curls

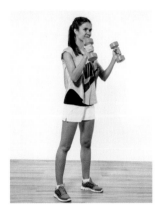

A standard exercise for bulging biceps. And remember, as always, the number of repetitions refers to just one side. Page 106.

Continue with:
Exercise 4, Seated row. ➡

Beginners 10 repetitions, Intermediates 15 repetitions, **Pros 20 repetitions**

4) Seated row (with band)

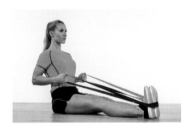

Works the shoulder muscles, back, and arms. Page 97.

Continue with:
Exercise 5, Ball crunches. ➡

Beginners 15 repetitions, Intermediates 20 repetitions, **Pros 25 repetitions**

5) Ball crunches

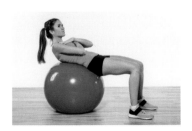

Crunches are a classic abdominal workout. The ball makes the exercise gentler on the back. Page 80.

Continue with:
Exercise 6, Upright row. ➡

Beginners 20 repetitions, Intermediates 30 repetitions, **Pros 40 repetitions**

6) Upright row

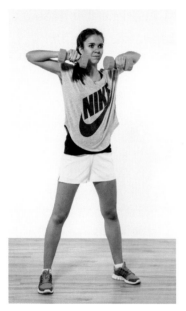

Ideal shoulder exercise – muscle soreness guaranteed! Make sure your movements are slow and controlled. Page 119.

Continue with:
Exercise 7, Squat - shoulder press. ➡

Beginners 10 repetitions, Intermediates 15 repetitions, **Pros 20 repetitions**

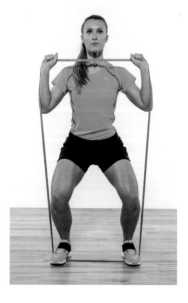

7) Squat – shoulder press

Works the entire body. The squat makes this extremely effective. Page 86.

Continue with:
Exercise 8, Forward ball roller. ➡

Beginners 5 repetitions, Intermediates 10 repetitions, **Pros 20 repetitions**

8) Forward ball roller

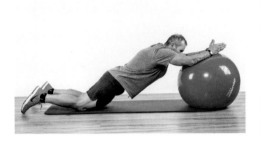

Works the core muscles. Be sure to maintain strong body tension and a straight back. Page 78.

Continue with:
Exercise 9, Chest flys on the stability ball. ➡

Beginners 10 repetitions, Intermediates 15 repetitions, **Pros 20 repetitions**

9) Chest flys on the stability ball

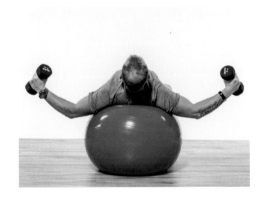

Homestretch! Here the focus is on chest and shoulders. However, lying on the ball also engages the core. Page 109.

Congratulations! Circuit completed!

Beginners 10 repetitions, Intermediates 15 repetitions, **Pros 20 repetitions**

Get fit with points! ✳✳✳

One set = 40 points
Two sets, 90 seconds break between sets = 70 points
Three sets, 90 seconds break between sets = 100 points
Four sets, 90 seconds break between sets = 150 points
Five sets = 90 seconds break between sets = 200 points

Tough guys - Tabata workout (Bodyweight)

Ladies, you can also get an amazing workout with this circuit. You will complete three Tabatas in a row – again 8 x 20 seconds load phase followed by a 10-second break. This time one Tabata consists of only two exercises which you will repeat for 4 x 20 seconds. That makes this circuit extremely tough. Have you managed to complete all three Tabatas once? Then you earned points for one set. After four sets, you have already earned the maximum number of 200 points.

Tabata A

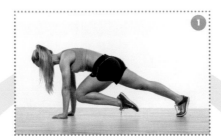

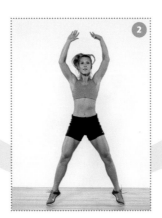

① Mountain climbers (4 x 20 seconds), page 131

② Jumping jacks (4 x 20 seconds), page 129

Tabata B

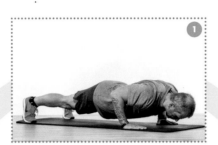

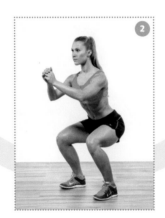

1 Classic pushups (4 x 20 seconds), page 136

2 Air squats (4 x 20 seconds), page 170

Tabata C

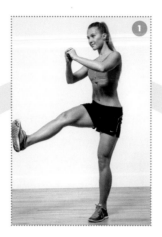

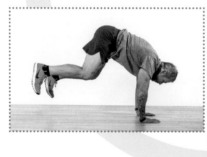

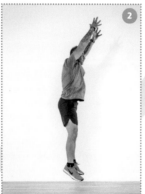

① Squat – kick (4 x 20 seconds), page 172

② Burpees (4 x 20 seconds), page 126

Get fit with points! ✳✳✳

One set = 40 points

Two sets, 90 seconds break between sets = 90 points

Three sets, 90 seconds break between sets = 145 points

Four sets, 90 seconds break between sets = 200 points

Early bird workout (Bodyweight, stability ball)

Working out right after waking up in the morning helps to get your circulation going, revive your spirits, and let you start your day with a wonderful sense of physical wellbeing. Admittedly, one has to get used to early morning workouts. But once you do, there is the risk of addiction. The following circuit only consists of six exercises, but works every muscle group. Complete a maximum of five sets which is worth 100 points.

1) Plank jacks

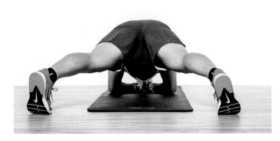

You are working the entire trunk, gluteals, shoulders, and legs. Page 157.

Continue with:
Exercise 2, Air squats. ➡

Beginners 10 repetitions, **Intermediates 20 repetitions**, **Pros 30 repetitions**

2) Air squats

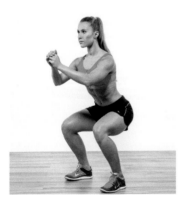

This is where you'll really wake up and crank up your circulation. Page 170.

Continue with:
Exercise 3, Jumping jacks. ➡

Beginners 10 repetitions, **Intermediates 20 repetitions**, **Pros 30 repetitions**

3) Jumping jacks

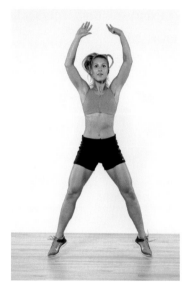

Another exercise that gets the entire body moving. Page 129.

Continue with:
Exercise 4, Russian twist (with ball). ➡

Beginners 15 repetitions, Intermediates 20 repetitions, **Pros 30 repetitions**

4) Russian twist (with ball)

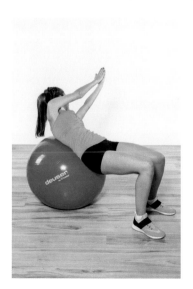

Now it's time to get the stability ball involved. You are primarily working the core muscles. As always, the number of repetitions refers to just one side - beginners lean 15 times to the left and 15 times to the right. Page 71.

Continue with:
Exercise 5, Double leg raises. ➡

Beginners 15 repetitions, Intermediates 20 repetitions, **Pros 30 repetitions**

5) Double leg raises

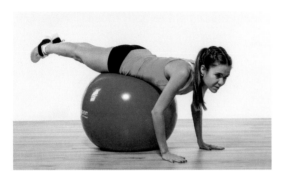

A lightweight exercise that primarily strengthens the lower back.

Continue with:
Exercise 6, Pushups on the ball. ➡

Beginners 10 repetitions, Intermediates 15 repetitions, **Pros 20 repetitions**

6) Pushups on the ball

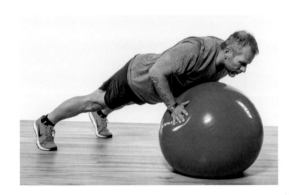

We'll finish with one more tough exercise. The ball's instability forces the upper body to work even harder. Page 70.

Beginners 5 repetitions, Intermediates 10 repetitions, **Pros 15 repetitions**

Get fit with points! ✳✳✳

One set = 10 points
Two sets, 90 seconds break between sets = 25 points
Three sets, 90 seconds break between sets = 45 points
Four sets, 90 seconds break between sets = 70 points
Five sets, 90 seconds break between sets = 100 points

Six-pack workout
(Bodyweight, stability ball, free weights)

If you have made summer vacation plans but don't have your beach body, the following circuit will burn your abs. You don't get a six-pack by just working your abs. You have to simultaneously burn fat so that your muscles become visible. Nevertheless, if you regularly focus on your core during your workouts, you will quickly see progress.

1) Boxer crunches

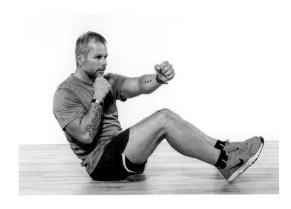

Everyone is familiar with crunches. In this variation, you get the shoulders involved by adding punches to the exercise. Page 160.

Continue with:
Exercise 2, Plank jacks. ➡

Beginners 10 repetitions, **Intermediates 20 repetitions**, **Pros 30 repetitions**

2) Plank jacks

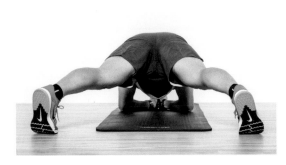

An excellent exercise for the entire core. And abductors and adductors are also working. Page 157.

Continue with:
Exercise 3, Jackknife with the ball. ➡

Beginners 10 repetitions, **Intermediates 20 repetitions**, **Pros 30 repetitions**

3) Jackknife with the ball

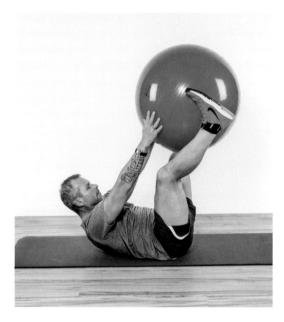

Suck it up! This exercise is definitely not for wimps! Make sure your movements are slow and controlled. Page 73.

Continue with:
Exercise 4, Swimmer. ➡

Beginners 10 repetitions, **Intermediates 20 repetitions**, **Pros 30 repetitions**

4) Swimmer

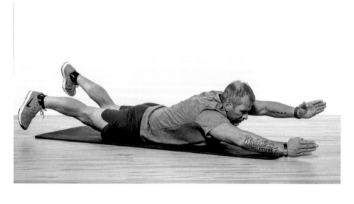

Extreme low-back workout. Maintain maximum body tension! Page 149.

Continue with:
Exercise 5, Crunches with free weights. ➡

Beginners 10 seconds, **Intermediates 20 seconds**, **Pros 30 seconds**

5) Crunches with free weights

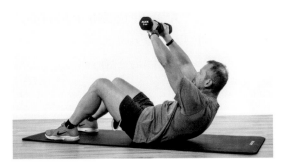

Extremely tough – for the belly, but the weights also work the shoulders. Page 122.

Continue with:
Exercise 6, Bilateral hip and trunk extension.
➡

Beginners 10 repetitions, Intermediates 20 repetitions, **Pros 30 repetitions**

6) Bilateral hip and trunk extension

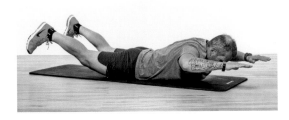

Time to work the abdominals' antagonist, the lower back. Page 155.

Continue with:
Exercise 7, Fingers to toes. ➡

Beginners 10 repetitions, Intermediates 20 repetitions, **Pros 30 repetitions**

7) Fingers to toes

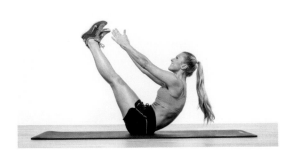

One of the toughest abdominal exercises overall. Page 154.

Continue with:
Exercise 8, Double leg raises. ➡

Beginners 10 repetitions, Intermediates 20 repetitions, **Pros 30 repetitions**

8) Double leg raises

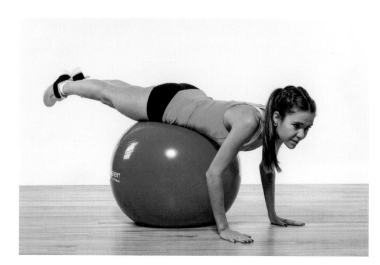

A gentle ending to this tough six-pack circuit. This one primarily works the lower back. Page 74.

Beginners 10 repetitions, Intermediates 20 repetitions, **Pros 30 repetitions**

Get fit with points! ✳✳✳
One set = 40 points
Two sets, 90 seconds break between sets = 80 points
Three sets, 90 seconds break between sets = 120 points
Four sets, 90 seconds break between sets = 160 points
Five sets, 90 seconds break between sets = 200 poin

Cardio workout (Bodyweight)

You don't feel like jogging regularly? You don't have to. If you just want to lose weight or work on a healthy fitness level, endurance-oriented bodyweight training is actually much more effective. The following circuit consists of five cardio exercises, each of which you should perform for 30-90 seconds at a time. You can take breaks of equal length in-between exercises. Can you do four sets? Congratulations, because then you deserve the maximum number of points!

1) Jumping jacks

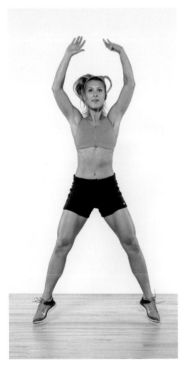

This classic at the start brings the entire body up to operating temperature. Page 129.

Break for 30, 60, or 90 seconds depending on your level and then continue with exercise 2: Butt kicks. ➡

Beginners 30 seconds, **Intermediates 60 seconds, Pros 90 seconds**

2) Butt kicks

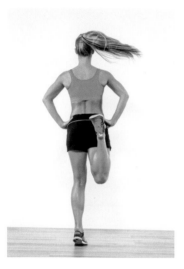

This gets pretty strenuous after a while. Next to endurance, this is also very good for the legs. Page 130.

Break for 30, 60, or 90 seconds depending on your level and continue with exercise 3: High knees. ➡

Beginners 30 seconds, **Intermediates 60 seconds**, **Pros 90 seconds**

3) High knees

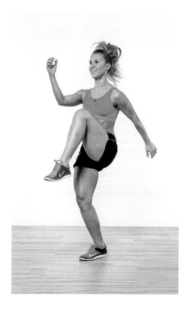

By now you should be reaching your limit. In the long, run high knees are a great fat killer. Page 128.

Break for 30, 60, or 90 seconds depending on your level and continue with exercise 4: Mountain climbers. ➡

Beginners 30 seconds, **Intermediates 60 seconds**, **Pros 90 seconds**

4) Mountain climbers

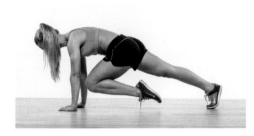

Are you cursing throughout this circuit? Suck it up and don't give up, no matter what! Your body will thank you. Page 131.

Break for 30, 60, or 90 seconds depending on your level and continue with exercise 5: Shadowboxing. ➡

Beginners 30 seconds, **Intermediates 60 seconds**, **Pros 90 seconds**

5) Shadowboxing

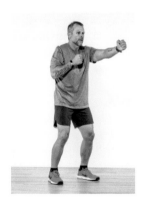

Now it's up to you how intensely you want to finish this circuit. The faster you bob and weave, the greater the challenge. Page 132.

Beginners 30 seconds, **Intermediates 60 seconds**, **Pros 90 seconds**

Wow, circuit completed! Take a 2-minute break – then start the second set!

Get fit with points! ✳✳✳
One set = 30 points
Two sets, 90 seconds break between sets = 70 points
Three sets, 90 seconds break between sets = 120 points
Four sets, 90 seconds break between sets = 200 points

Hardcore workout (Bodyweight)

The ultimate circuit for the toughest of the toughest. This is for all those who don't just want to hit their limit but want to push beyond it. It is for those who really want to torture themselves and see what their body is capable of.

You will complete 10 exercises – each for one minute. You can rest exactly 30 seconds between exercises. This time there are no levels.

1) Mountain climbers

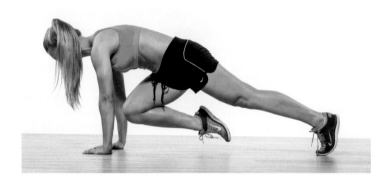

Page 131

60 seconds

2) Burpees

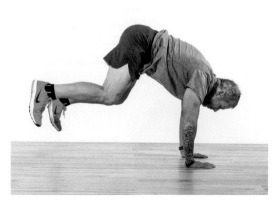

Page 126

60 seconds

3) High knees

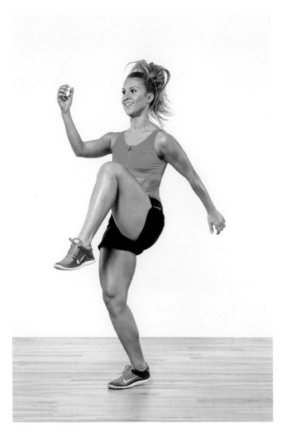

Page 128

60 seconds

4) Triangle pushups

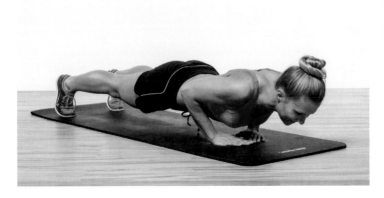

Page 137

60 seconds

5) Jump lunges

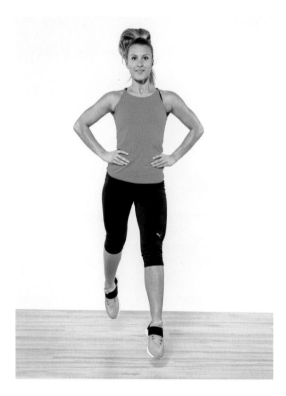

Page 173

60 seconds

6) Fingers to toes

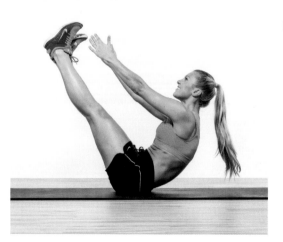

Page 154

60 seconds

7) Bridge

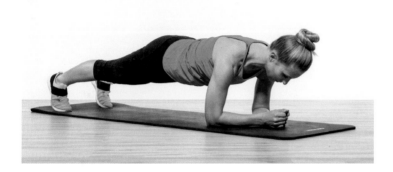

Page 164

60 seconds

8) Jump squats

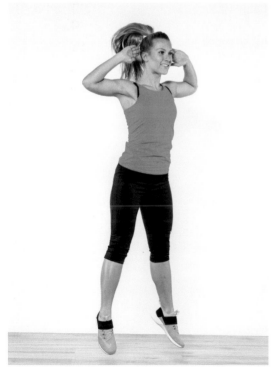

Page 174

60 seconds

9) Jumping jacks

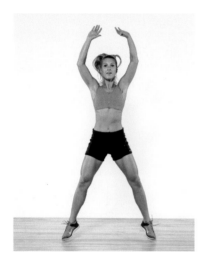

Page 129

(60 seconds)

10) Helicopter reverse curls

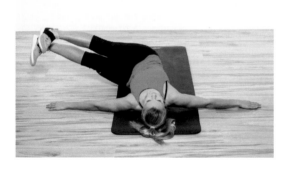

Page 162

60 seconds

Get fit with points! ✳✳✳
One set = 60 points
Two sets, 90 seconds break between sets = 130 points
Three sets, 90 seconds break between sets = 200 points
Four sets, 90 seconds break between sets = 300 points

Gentle back workout (Bodyweight, stability ball)

Back problems are extremely common but spinal problems can easily be prevented. When you regularly work the core and thereby strengthen the core muscles, you create the basis for a healthier back.

1) Ball crunches

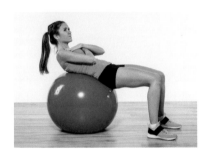

Let's start with an abdominal exercise. The soft ball makes the exercise easy on the back. Page 80.

Continue with:
Exercise 2, Double leg raises. ➡

Beginners 10 repetitions, Intermediates 20 repetitions, **Pros 30 repetitions**

2) Double leg raises

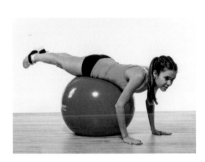

You will need the stability ball for this exercise as well. The exercise strengthens the lower back. Page 74.

Continue with:
Exercise 3, The bug. ➡

Beginners 10 repetitions, Intermediates 20 repetitions, **Pros 30 repetitions**

3) The bug

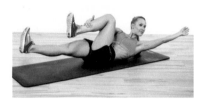

Now back to working the belly. Maintain maximum body tension. Page 152.

Continue with:
Exercise 4, Prone leg raises. ➡

Beginners 10 repetitions, **Intermediates 20 repetitions**, **Pros 30 repetitions**

4) Prone leg raises

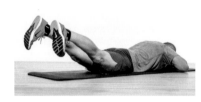

Effective for the lower back and can be done by just about anyone. As an alternative, you can raise the legs one at a time. Page 151.
Continue with:
Exercise 5, Russian twist (with ball). ➡

Beginners 10 repetitions, **Intermediates 20 repetitions**, **Pros 30 repetitions**

5) Russian twist

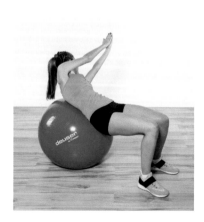

You should already be familiar with this exercise. You will primarily work the oblique abdominal muscles. Page 71.

Continue with:
Exercise 6, Moving side plank. ➡

Beginners 10 repetitions, **Intermediates 20 repetitions**, **Pros 30 repetitions**

6) Moving side plank

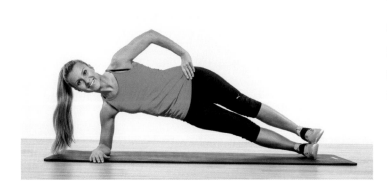

The final exercise in this circuit. As always, the repetitions refer to just one side – for instance left, then right. Page 165.

Beginners 10 repetitions, Intermediates 20 repetitions, **Pros 30 repetitions**

Get fit with points! ✳✳✳
One set = 10 points
Two sets, 90 seconds break between sets = 25 points
Three sets, 90 seconds break between sets = 45 points
Four sets, 90 seconds break between sets = 70 points
Five sets, 90 seconds break between sets = 100 points

Resistance band Tabata

We will wrap up the circuit chapter by going back to the exercise bands one more time. You will complete three different Tabatas, meaning you will again complete 8 x 20-second load phases with 10 seconds of rest after each of those phases. Here, one Tabata consists of two exercises. The focus is on upper body and legs.

Beginner version:
Alternate between exercise 1 and exercise 2 (20 seconds each) with 10 seconds rest in-between.

Intermediate version:
2 x 20 seconds exercise 1, 2 x 20 seconds exercise 2, 2 x 20 seconds exercise 1, 2 x 20 seconds exercise 2.

Pro version:
4 x 20 seconds exercise 1, 4 x 20 seconds exercise 2.

Tabata A

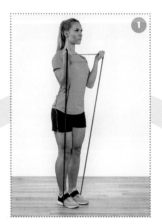

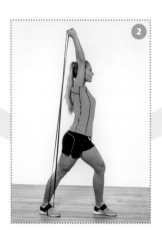

1 Bicep curls, page 91

2 Triceps press, page 93

Tabata B

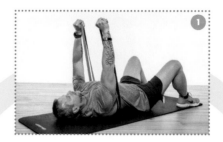

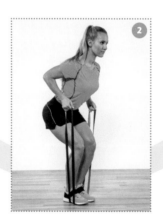

1. Reclined chest press, page 90

2. Double-arm bent-over row, page 96

Tabata C

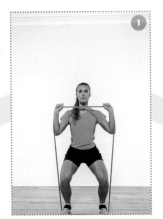

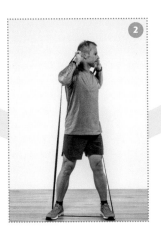

1. Squat – shoulder press, page 86

2. Squat with rotation, page 101

10 NUTRITION:
FUEL FOR THE BODY

Would you put old diesel fuel into a sleek sports car? Probably not, because you would worry about causing damage to the engine. I regularly ask myself why most people approach their diet so terribly. Many still believe that they can tackle their personal Mount. Everest while eating industrially mass-produced processed foods, meat from CAFOs, and junk food. The consequences, particularly long-term health damage, of unhealthy and in some cases contaminated foods have long been scientifically proven. There is now even an increased amount of media coverage on the subject.

In recent decades, excess weight, especially in Europe and the US, has become a serious problem. According to various studies, more than 1 in 2 Germans carry too much weight, and every fourth German suffers from resulting serious health problems. In the US, every third person suffers from obesity. What is worse is that this disease has frightening effects on human health. Nearly 50% of adults in the US are diabetic or pre-diabetic.

This is without a doubt the result of an unhealthy diet.

Our insurance companies are having to bear the increasing costs because so many people are poisoning their body with sugary foods every day and as a result, getting sick. The fact that a bad diet is the cause for many illnesses is just as indisputable as the opposite finding that a good diet can have a healing and preventative effect. There are few illnesses that cannot be at least mitigated by adjusting the individual diet plan.

I have already talked about the cornerstones of a balanced diet −proteins, good and bad fats, as well as carbohydrates and some supplements- in our first book (*Bodyweight Training mit Mike Diehl*). I explained that scientific research today is so extensive and fast, that the subject of nutrition continues to develop into an increasingly complex field. New, groundbreaking research findings are presented nearly every week, resulting in new nutritional and dietary trends.

For example, around 10% of Germans banned foods containing gluten from their diet, in spite of the fact that only 1% at most actually suffer from a gluten intolerance (celiac disease).

Vegetarian or even vegan cookbooks continue to move up on bestseller lists as the market for dietary advice continues to expand. I personally value a balanced diet that includes meat because it contains important proteins. But it is up to the individual whether or not he chooses to consume low-quality products that contain harmful substances.

Perhaps the better choice is to eat meat less often and instead accept the higher cost of organically grown products. Or another option is completely abstaining from animal products for ethical reasons. There is no one-size-fits-all solution.

Fresh fruit and vegetables should be on the menu every day. But here, too, it is important to note that many products sold in supermarkets have been sprayed with pesticides in order to keep them edible for longer, and are thereby contaminated. It is important to also check the origins of the product. And it is common knowledge that whole-grain products such as brown rice and dark bread are much healthier than foods that contain wheat.

Unaltered natural, so-called *good fats* are essential to a balanced diet. They are the number one energy supplier, providing twice as much energy (calories) as the same quantity of protein or carbohydrates. Lean, protein-rich poultry and fish are equally as important. We now also know that many types of fish, particularly farm-raised varieties, are not nearly as healthy as they were once believed to be.

More and more studies show that salmon and trout often contain harmful substances, resulting from contaminated fish food that we ingest with the fish, which over time can promote certain types of cancer, heart ailments or diabetes. It is therefore extremely important to carefully check the origins of our food and develop awareness for what and how much we can in good conscience put into our bodies.

If you would like to learn more about nutrition, I would suggest reading some relevant practical guidebooks. A fitness book that focuses on a large selection of exercises, workouts, and circuits realistically does not offer such extensive and complex explanations as a book whose subject matter is strictly nutritional advice. This chapter on nutrition on the following pages focuses on questions about the correct use of supplements, meaning the necessary dietary supplements for an athlete.

Dietary supplements – important or a rip-off?

Few topics in competitive sports are as hotly debated as the need for dietary supplements. I receive questions daily on my social media channels or via email from athletes that want to know which supplements are highly recommended, which protein powder is best for muscle growth, and which products will promote fat burning or help to accelerate regeneration.

One thing is clear, however, each year the dietary supplement industry grosses unbelievable amounts of money with the products not meeting the advertised promises made to customers. In fact, I maintain that many of the supplements on the market are completely ineffective and yet the manufacturers continue to profit from this.

If you research online or look at trade magazines, you will be inundated with product recommendations and will see many more ads for dietary supplements than for exercise equipment – because the industry continues to grow.

Should you therefore completely forgo dietary supplements? I don't think so. But I do, however, suggest that you find out which supplements would truly be beneficial to your goals, whether the effectiveness of the product has been scientifically proven. When in doubt, it is best to consult nutritional experts or fitness coaches that you trust.

The fact is that a balanced diet is the basis for a healthy body. Supplements can be beneficial for optimizing your diet and getting slightly more energy from your body when you exercise. But they are no substitute for a healthy diet.

The pyramid illustrates the important difference between a high-quality and healthy diet that must always be the focus, and supplementation that only occurs at the top.

Which basic supplements are beneficial?

For ambitious athletes looking for optimal performance capacity as well as quick regeneration and prevention of infections, I primarily recommend the following supplements:

- Vitamin D
- Omega-3 fatty acids (fish oil)
- Magnesium
- Zinc
- Vitamin C

Vitamin D deficiency has become very common. Today's life style, that has us increasingly tied down to computers and cell phones, keeping many of us from occasionally catching a little sunshine, is largely to blame. But vitamin D isn't just produced in the skin from the sunshine, it can also be derived from our diet or supplements.

Vitamin D supplementation can have advantages such as: increased mental capacity, healthier bones, a stronger immune system, an increased sense of wellbeing, and a decreased risk of cancer, heart disease, diabetes, multiple sclerosis, high blood pressure, or osteoporosis. Many autoimmune diseases often seem to be associated with a vitamin-D deficiency.

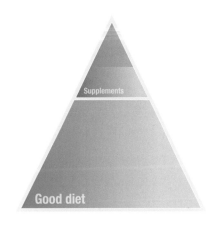

The correct dosage is complicated and is dependent on how much vitamin D can already be produced in the skin from sun exposure. This means that the seasons also play a role. In summer, our entire vitamin-D requirement can generally be met with sunshine. This is, however, not the case in the winter time. Many experts recommend an average of 2000 to 2500 IE per day during the winter months. However, blanket statements are problematic, and I therefore always recommend talking to a doctor or pharmacist.

Here is what you need to know. Vitamin D preparations should be taken with a little fat. I recommend taking it in the morning along with **omega-3 fatty acids**. These are particularly important. Due to today's diet in Western Europe, we tend to consume too much omega-6 fatty acids (in animal and plant fats) and too little omega-3 fatty acids. Their positive effects on the body's exercise-induced inflammatory processes have long been proven in different studies.

The different effects of omega-3 fatty acids (promotes fat burning, anti-inflammatory, promotes muscle growth, lowers blood pressure, promotes insulin sensitivity, increases brain function, protects from heart ailments and arteriosclerosis, etc.) are achieved through increased cell wall elasticity. They attach themselves along with other fatty acids, and the higher the share of omega-3, the more flexible the cell membrane becomes. What matters is the balanced ratio of omega-6 to omega-3 fatty acids. The German Nutrition Society, Inc. recommends a ratio of 5:1. In reality, it is often 7:1 or even higher.

Different experts recommend a supplementary dose of two capsules a day (2g omega-3). I take one in the morning and one at night. Here, too, individual advice is recommended, also with respect to choice of preparation.

Foods high in omega-6 fatty acids: e.g. Sunflower oil, soybean oil, Chia seeds, tuna fish, liver sausage, pork, chicken, beef, salmon, mackerel.

Foods high in omega-3 fatty acids: e.g. flaxseed oil, rapeseed oil, Chia seeds, salmon, herring, tuna fish, sprat, mackerel.

An additional **magnesium** supplement is essential for athletes. Because of today's diet, magnesium deficiency is also very common. That is why this essential mineral belongs on the list of basis supplements.

Magnesium is known as the anti-stress mineral because it prevents excessive brain stimulation. It also improves insulin sensitivity and has a positive effect on blood pressure. Magnesium is also linked to the mind. People suffering from depression or learning disabilities are often diagnosed with a magnesium deficiency. But it primarily has a relaxing and anti-inflammatory effect.

Many athletes suffer from muscle cramps after arduous competitions, or just in general after intense physical activity because their magnesium requirements are no longer being met and the muscles are not receiving an adequate energy supply. Experts recommend an average of 400 mg per day of elemental magnesium (equals approx. 2.6 g of magnesium citrate).

Foods containing magnesium: e.g. pumpkin seeds (approx. 530 mg/100 g), flaxseed (approx. 350 mg/100 g), peanuts (approx. 160 mg/100 g), cocoa (approx. 400 mg/100 g), soybeans (approx. 220 mg/100 g), sunflower seeds (approx. 420 mg/100 g).

Zinc is an essential trace element. It is vital to our health and plays a role in many metabolic reactions. Zinc is important for growth, the skin, insulin storage, sperm production, and the immune system. Zinc strengthens the body's immune defenses. It possesses anti-viral properties and is therefore considered a panacea for the prevention of colds, or at least for shortening their duration.

The consequences of a zinc deficiency can be many: hair loss, chapped and dry skin, diminished wound repair, skin infections, growth disturbance in children, loss of appetite, impotence, weakened immune system, and a fundamentally limited performance capacity.

Athletes in particular often have a zinc deficiency because the trace mineral is excreted in sweat.

Since our bodies don't have any storage space, it is important to ingest zinc on a daily basis in our food. The German Society for Nutritional Medicine and Diet, Inc. recommends a daily zinc intake of approx. 15 mg, and as much as 25 mg for pregnant women and nursing mothers. Physical exertion and stress also increase the requirement, so athletes in particular should ensure a sufficient zinc intake.

Foods containing zinc: e.g. oysters, beef, ocean fish, seafood, eggs, whole-grain products.

Vitamin C supplements and protects zinc's numerous and health-protecting metabolic effects. It increases the effects of zinc. That is why prefabricated compounds from the pharmacy often contain both substances.

Which special supplements are advisable?

So-called *special supplementation* is much more specific than basis supplements. They are geared to the athlete's specific goals like building muscle, burning fat, or an overall increase in performance. Ambitious athletes, and particularly those looking for significant muscle growth can't do without an increased **protein intake**.

When I talk to my athletes, I often notice that many people don't differentiate between the types of proteins that they consume. Be it meat, eggs, fish, cheese, or legumes – all of these foods are high in protein and seem to serve their purpose. But most people forget that not all protein sources are automatically effective, for instance with respect to muscle growth.

I like to compare the human body to a house during the construction of which we think deeply about which materials we need and most importantly, which products are important long-term. Just like a house, our bodies also needs the appropriate "building materials."

The richest protein sources for healthy muscle growth are animal proteins, meaning milk, eggs, fish or meat. For competitive athletes and those working towards becoming one,

protein from the tin also plays an important role, because no one can eat meat and fish by the pound, or consume dozens of eggs.

We differentiate between **whey** and **casein** protein powder. Both types of protein are present in milk and are thus considered natural, not artificial. Milk generally consists of about 80% casein and 20% whey. Both types are nutritious and nutrient-rich. However, due to their different properties with respect to the metabolic process, both have advantages and disadvantages. While whey and casein come from the same source, the amino acids that they contain are released into the blood at different rates– whey faster and casein slower. I therefore like to call whey a sports car and casein a tractor.

That doesn't mean we should always prefer the speedster. I regularly use both whey and casein. I usually consume whey right after working out to ensure a quick protein supply, and I frequently have a casein shake as a meal substitute.

You can think of whey as a kind of raiding squad that gets to where it is needed extremely quickly, namely the cells, but also disappearing again just as fast. Casein on the other hand has an anti-catabolic effect because it is digested slowly and ensures a steady inflow of amino acids. Compared to whey concentrates, casein offers about three times the amount of calcium. Calcium is responsible for our muscle contractions and is a coenzyme in blood clotting.

In addition to protein powders, a special **creatine** supplement is another dietary supplement option. The name comes from the Greek word *"kreas,"* meaning meat. Creatine is an endogenous substance that primarily resides in the muscles and is part of the energy supply system.

Creatine is produced in the kidneys, the pancreas, and the liver. It consists of three different amino acids. The amount of creatine in the human body varies and is dependent on age, gender, and genetic predisposition. Diet also plays a critical role. Athletes that eat large quantities of meat are shown to have a higher creatine level than vegetarians.

Herring has an extremely high creatine content – 8-10 g per kg! Creatine's chief virtue is that, as an energy supplier, it contributes to the synthesis of adenosine triphosphate (ATP), thereby facilitating muscle contraction. The more creatine available in a muscle cell, the longer the muscles can generate maximum performance. Creatine facilitates increased performance capacity during short-term loads like strength and speed-strength training, or sprints. It also boosts regeneration, which is why bodybuilders and endurance athletes often use creatine as a dietary supplement.

The more often and the harder we work out, the higher our creatine requirement and consumption. This is why many athletes swear by supplements because their effectiveness has been scientifically proven via many studies. Experts generally recommend that competitive athletes get 3 grams of additional creatine per day.

L-arginine is another special supplement that I recommend to many athletes. I also regularly take this myself. L-arginine is considered a semi-essential amino acid. This means that the human body can, to some extent, produce it with a healthy metabolism. However, the body's production doesn't always meet the daily requirements.

Essential amino acids are those the body cannot produce on its own and must therefore be absorbed from food. The body produces non-essential amino acids.

What does L-arginine do? It facilitates better circulation. L-arginine is present in hemoglobin that supplies the organs, muscles, and skin with oxygen. It increases blood flow in the veins and arteries, and regulates oxygen transport. The effects of L-arginine are also said to control high blood pressure. Other important effects of L-arginine are improved muscle growth and faster regeneration. The increased oxygen supply makes muscle fibers more resilient and minimizes muscle disorders. L-arginine is also said to have a positive effect on our short and long-term memory, and a palliative effect on Alzheimer's and dementia.

Positive effects can also be ascertained in cases of: stroke, multiple sclerosis, rheumatoid arthritis, allergies, depression, weak bladder, osteoporosis, etc.

For L-arginine to have a lasting effect, it should be taken permanently. With regular ingestion, initial effects are generally noticeable within 4-8 weeks.

L-arginine can be taken in powder-form and can be mixed with cocoa or tea. Another alternative are capsules and tablets. I personally take 4.5 g of L-arginine daily. However, many experts recommend a lower dose. The body does generally tolerate larger amounts without any problems or side effects but I recommend seeking advice from nutritional experts or physicians.

Foods high in L-arginine: oats, walnuts, soybeans, wheat germ, peanuts.

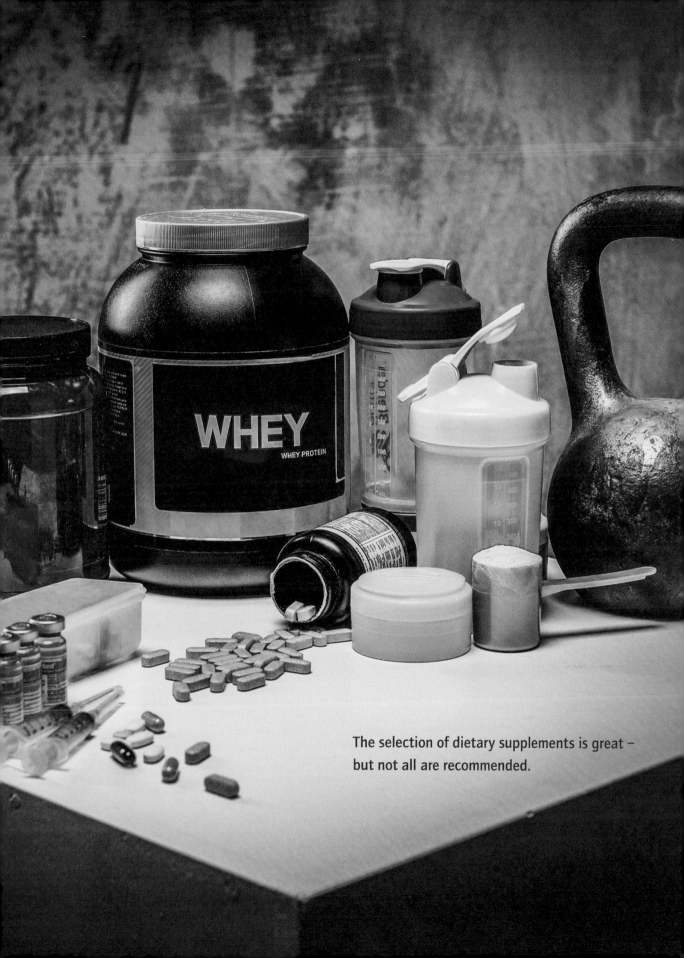

The selection of dietary supplements is great – but not all are recommended.

11 Q & A: EVERYTHING YOU ALWAYS WANTED TO KNOW ABOUT FITNESS TRAINING

Does a protein-rich diet help you lose weight?

Protein-rich foods like poultry, fish, buttermilk or yoghurt, satiate us for a particularly long time without being extremely high in calories or fat. Moreover, there are different studies that verify that proteins stimulate the release of satiety hormones in the body. That means we are less hungry, and therefore consume less food.

Protein-rich foods should therefore often be on the menu. There are now different studies that prove that a low-fat diet isn't necessarily a low-calorie diet. Many low-fat products contain lots of sugar or carbohydrates. Therefore, these foods often have a higher calorie content than high-fat foods.

And at this time I would like to correct another misconception. Regardless of what advertisers want us to believe, light products do not help you lose weight! They contain large amounts of sugar or sugar substitutes that get us used to the sugary taste and cause long-term addiction. Hands off!

Does eating at night make you fat?

This is another myth that has long been disproven. It used to be a common belief that the later you eat, the higher the risk of gaining weight and getting fat. Today we know that the deciding factor is actually our daily calorie consumption and the amount of exercise we get. Thus there is no argument against a relaxed dinner, other than the fact that many people don't sleep well on a full stomach.

What are the advantages of regular strength training?

Strength training builds muscle. Over time our body becomes tighter, firmer, and more robust. Strength training also helps you to lose weight. On the one hand, you burn fat and build muscle. On the other hand, muscle consumes energy when we move, even when we are just sitting on the couch. The more muscle mass we have, the more calories we burn. While we also gain muscle with endurance exercise, it is less pronounced. In addition to our muscles, strength training also strengthens tendons, ligaments, and bones. By doing strength exercises, we can prevent back pain osteoporosis, among other things.

How important is endurance training?

A balanced exercise routine includes endurance, strength, and mobility training, for instance in the form of stretching. People who only focus on building muscle are neglecting their cardio-vascular system. And people who only work on endurance build little muscle that helps to burn calories and protect us from weight gain.

Should I cool down after working out?

The answer is an unequivocal "yes!" A *cool-down* is just as important as a warm-up before every training unit. A successful cool-down has a psychological and physiological effect on the body. During a workout, the cardio-vascular system works particularly hard. If the exertion ends abruptly, the body doesn't get a chance to gradually power down. The muscles also need a slow relaxation phase. An effective cool-down loosens up the muscles and allows the entire body to regenerate.

I always tell my clients that a good and healthy workout challenges the body and the mind. This outlook allows us athletes to stay in control and achieve personal best performances again and again. In my opinion, relaxing with a cool-down is essential to finding our way back to everyday life after a workout. It is a way to gain a fresh perspective and the ability to tackle subsequent tasks with a lighter heart. That is particularly important for a spontaneous workout such as at the workplace, which then requires our focus to immediately shift onto other things.

Why is the warm-up so important?

Always remember one of my most important principles. Working out is not supposed to be a burden, it should be pleasurable. A short, but effective warm-up affects the body and the mind in a complex way. The warm-up is an optimal preparation of all body systems (including the head!) for increased activity as well as injury prevention. We should not view the warm-up as a burdensome duty but as the first important step towards better health. Warming up should create the desire for more exercise!

For example

a) **The cardiovascular system:** the heart beats faster and more blood circulates through the body because the blood reservoirs (for instance the liver) release reserves. This supplies the working muscles with more nutrients and oxygen. At the same time, the removal of metabolic waste products improves, preventing overacidification of the muscles.

b) **Joints and ligaments:** the body produces more synovial fluid, which increases the amount of cartilage, allowing for better buffering against pressure on the cartilage generated by athletic activity. Tendons and ligaments get more elastic with a rise in body temperature.

c) **The mind:** warming up improves an athlete's concentration and cognitive ability, making it possible for the athlete to read certain situations (e.g. suddenly appearing obstacles while running) more quickly. They will also better recognize possible injury risks. Optimal warm-ups also improve motivation for the subsequent athletic performance, they loosen up cramped muscles, and reduce potential reluctance.

That means skipping the warm-up won't distinguish you as a tough guy. It actually lays the foundation for a beneficial athletic activity.

Do you have questions for Mike Diehl?
You can contact him anytime on his website www.mike-diehl.de, or on our Facebook platform "Dein Fitness Coach – Mike Diehl."

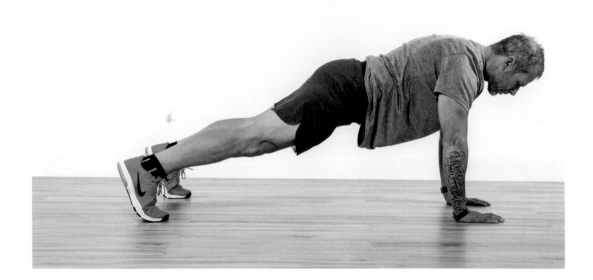

APPENDIX

References

Löffler G., Petrides P., Heinrich P. (2007). *Biochemie & Pathobiochemie* (8. Auflage). Heidelberg: Springer Medizin Verlag.

Bertram, O. (2014). *Das Men's Health Workout ohne Geräte* (2. Auflage). München: Südwest Verlag.

Diehl, M., Grewe, F. (2017): *Bodyweight Training mit Mike Diehl* (1. Auflage). Aachen: Meyer & Meyer Verlag.

Herzner, S. (12. Mai 2015). *Apotheken Umschau: Was sind eigentlich Fette?* Baierbrunn bei München Wort & Photo Verlag Konradshöhe GmbH & Co. KG.

Additional online sources

www.schmidt-sports.de

www.gymnastikball-sitzball.de

Photo credits

Photos:

Stefan von Stengel

Interior and Cover Design: Annika Naas
Layout: Guido Maetzing
Managing Editor: Elizabeth Evans
Copyeditor: Qurratulain Zaheer

THE AUTHORS

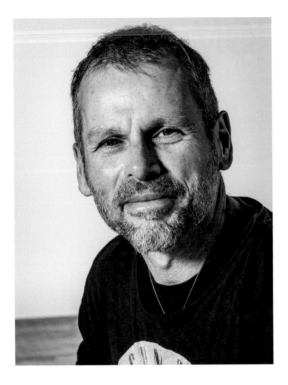

Mike Diehl

Mike Diehl lives in Cologne, Germany. He is a certified trainer for competitive sports as well as health, fitness, and sports rehabilitation. He is also a mental and relaxation coach, as well as a physical fitness coach for the German Army. As a soldier, he spent years on active duty with the Special Forces. Since 2007, he has been the fitness coach for the German Fed-Cup team (Ladies National Tennis Team), where he trains top players like Angelique Kerber or Julia Görges, a. o. Diehl works as a fitness trainer for the tennis association Mittelrhein. In the past, he trained the Fortuna Düsseldorf soccer players and the DEG Metro Starts ice hockey team.

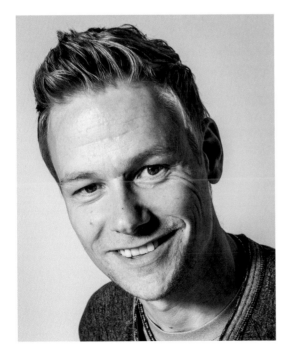

Felix Grewe

Felix Grewe lives in Hamburg, Germany. He studied sports writing and sports management in college and for many years worked in the field as a reporter for the trade journal *tennis MAGAZIN*. Today, he is head of media and public relations at the German Tennis Federation. He is an expert in tennis and physical fitness and helps to put Mike Diehl's exercises and methods into words. He has been using the Coach's plans for years in his own regular workouts.

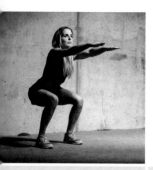

MORE FROM

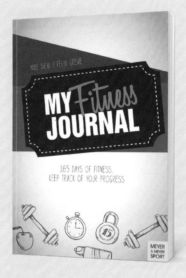

208 p., b/w

Hardcover

6.5 x 9.25"

ISBN: 9781782551294

$9.95 US

Diehl | Grewe

My Fitness Journal

Put structure into your workouts! Write down your fitness sessions and weaknesses, your sporting goals, and your eating habits. Make regular progress checks, including progress photos, to keep track of how much your fitness level is advancing. Compare your workouts to reach your goals faster.

◗ You will find a bonus preview on the following pages.

MEYER & MEYER

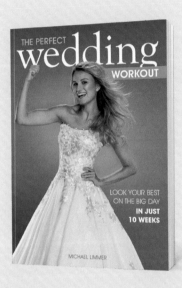

216 p., in color

215 photos + illus.

Paperback

6.5 x 9.25"

ISBN: 9781782551461

$16.95 US

Limmer

The Perfect Wedding Workout

This book is the perfect fitness program for every bride who wants to look her best on her wedding day, and it only takes 10 weeks. It provides an at-home fitness program that is designed specifically for the needs of the bride-to-be. Within it are the secrets of a target-oriented diet and it also includes professional beauty tips for a perfect wedding look.

MEYER & MEYER
Sport
Von-Coels-Str. 390
52080 Aachen, Germany

Phone   02 41 - 9 58 10 - 13
Fax   02 41 - 9 58 10 - 10
E-Mail   sales@m-m-sports.com
Website   www.thesportspublisher.com

All books available as e-books.

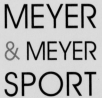

MY *Fitness* JOURNAL

MY PERSONAL FITNESS JOURNAL

Name:

Address:

Telephone:

E-Mail:

Weight:

Body-fat percentage/Waist measurement:

Height:

Training start date:

My fitness level:

| 1 | 2 | 3 | 4 | 5 | 6 | 7 | 8 | 9 | 10 |

My physical strengths:

My physical weaknesses:

My training motto:

So I prefer to train:

My training goals for the next 365 days:

In three months I will …

_____

_____

In six months I will …

_____

_____

In nine months I will …

_____

_____

In twelve months I will …

_____

_____

My photo from   .   . 20

Place full-body shot here

My Body

What is *acceptance*? It is the ability to recognize the reality of your body's problem zones. Be honest with yourself and accurately analyze what circumstances and living habits have led to your present fitness level. Regularly check up on your progress to see if there is change or stagnation in your fitness level.

In the following spaces, you can place a photo of you every three months. Use these photos to check your progress. They can be full-body images or only photos of your problem zones. At the end of your training year, look again at these photos to see how your hard work has paid off.

Photo 1:

My comments:

Photo 2:

My comments: